The Creation of Aesthetic Plastic Surgery

The Creation of Aesthetic Plastic Surgery

Edited by
Mario González-Ulloa

With 99 Figures

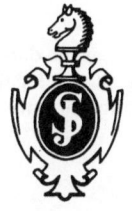

Springer Science+Business Media, LLC

Mario González-Ulloa
Centro Medico Dalinde
Mexico City, Mexico D.F.

Library of Congress Cataloging-in-Publication Data
Main entry under title:
The Creation of aesthetic plastic surgery.
  "These articles have appeared previously in Aesthetic plastic surgery":—Verso of t.p.
  Contents: The development of aesthetic plastic surgery / Blair O. Rogers—The history of blepharoplasty to correct blepharochalasis / Kathryn L. Stephenson—The history of rhytidectomy / Mario González-Ulloa—[etc.]
  1. Surgery, Plastic—Addresses, essays, lectures. I. González-Ulloa, Mario.
RD118.C74   1985   617'.95   85-17290

These articles have appeared previously in *Aesthetic Plastic Surgery*.

9 8 7 6 5 4 3 2 1

ISBN 978-0-387-96218-4   ISBN 978-1-4757-4319-7 (eBook)
DOI 10.1007/978-1-4757-4319-7

Foreword

In the turmoil of everyday activity, when few surgeons have time or energy for bibliographic research, the wonderful history of human endeavor runs the risk of remaining buried in libraries.

Several years ago, a small group of enthusiasts was gathered together by Mario González-Ulloa to write the history of Aesthetic Plastic Surgery. There was the feeling among them that experience and knowledge should be shared by all those who practice this art and this science, and that its creation and progress would be alive and present with a chronicle of this surgical specialty.

Their chapters have been written. These chapters have appeared in *Aesthetic Plastic Surgery*, but they are now collected in book form, and the individual style of each author has been preserved. It is a thrilling story. It is a compact information. Let it be our stepping-stone project in which past, present, and future are fused into one.

Jack E. Davis
Past President of ISAPS

Preface

History is a narration of facts, a description of how individuals gave meaning to facts, and an account of how human beings made facts a reality. Nothing is more fascinating than the study of man and his circumstances, because one has a direct bearing on the other. Through meaningful interaction the two can impregnate each other with an idea and give it life, creating a new concept, a new attitude, or even a new and different trend in the course of history. Thus, from people's desire to possess beauty, man has created new means for acquiring that sought after beauty. These means, in turn, have broken open whole new spheres of insight which push knowledge forward into unexplored fields of specialization, offering individuals formerly unknown options in that everlasting search.

The Creation of Aesthetic Plastic Surgery is a story of discovery. It describes how men explored and charted the realm of possibilities, bringing into existence new activities which today—in our present age—constitute an integrated geographical guide to the possible.

Many creative surgeons participated in creating the basis of the idea and the structure of the possibilities. They were followed by others who, like decorating the proverbial Christmas tree, have put their little glowing ornament in place. Who put the original Christmas tree in place? Who continued to decorate it while a new tree (another ideology) was being prepared? These questions go to the heart and purpose of this narration of facts. A logical consequence of the decorating process would be to make sure the tree did not become confused with or take on the name of any one of the ornaments. Nor should anyone reinvent an already developed process simply because he ignores the facts concerning previous discoveries.

The Creation of Aesthetic Plastic Surgery has been prepared by a team of individuals who readily responded to my call. They have worked together to create an historical basis for our specialized field. Some of them have worked over a period of many years gathering the materials which have made this editorial collection possible. In alphabetical order they are: Jack E. Davis, Jean Pierre Lalardrie, Frank McDowell, Roger Mouly, Paule Regnault, Blair O. Rogers. and Kathryn L. Stephenson.

The decision to publish this collection of articles in *Aesthetic Plastic Surgery,* the organ of the International Society of Aesthetic Plastic Surgery, was very carefully thought through. This is the first Aesthetic Surgery journal in the world. It is also the magazine which best reaches the individuals who most need this information. Furthermore, our decision is meant as a gesture of brotherhood from this team which has worked so laboriously to contribute a body of knowledge to a field which has been so controversial and misunderstood in the past.

Publication of this work in *Aesthetic Plastic Surgery* did not preclude its publishing in book form. Quite the contrary: our intention has always been to have the articles appear in this journal and then to publish them in the form of a reference book. This will give the scholar an opportunity to collect the history of his own times and endow himself with an accumulative education, thus giving form and substance to his experience.

While offering my congratulations to the colleagues who so willingly and effectively responded to my call, I must also express my appreciation to the editor, Blair Rogers, for his gracious understanding of our objectives and his help in giving a material expression to those objectives. To all of my colleagues I say, "Thank you." To the reader I say, "I trust you will find in this history an echo of your own creative drives. I hope you will use this narrative as a magnifying glass to augment and more clearly focus your own possibilities."

Mario González-Ulloa

Contents

Aesthetic Plastic Surgery 1:3-24, 1976
© 1976 by Springer-Verlag New York Inc.

The Development of Aesthetic Plastic Surgery: A History

Blair O. Rogers M.D.

New York, New York

"Do you set down your name in the scroll of youth, that are written down old with all the characters of age? Have you not a moist eye, a dry hand, a yellow cheek, a white beard, a decreasing leg, an increasing belly? Is not your voice broken, your wind short, your chin double, your wit single, and every part about you blasted with antiquity? And will you yet call yourself young?"

William Shakespeare
Henry IV, Part II, 2, 204 (62)

ABSTRACT / Aesthetic plastic surgery had its origins, probably with Dieffenbach, in the mid-1800's. In its earliest stages great use was made of external incisions in the facial region, which were obvious to the casual observer. Yet the true beginning of aesthetic plastic surgery as we know it today, was not until 1887, when John Orlando Roe introduced an intranasal corrective operation on the nose. From that time onward, aesthetic plastic surgery developed in a fascinating manner over the subsequent decades to become the fine scientific art we take for granted today.

Our modern definition of the scope of aesthetic (cosmetic) surgery more often than not concerns itself with the idea that this surgery is chiefly performed on the face and neck, and then to a much lesser degree on the breast region, and finally to an even smaller degree on the abdomen, buttock, and thigh regions. The purpose of this article will be to review briefly the beginnings of aesthetic surgery as we know it today, and because of the historic nature of things, it will deal largely and specifically with aesthetic surgery of the facial region. Subsequent articles in this new journal will describe the historic development of aesthetic breast, abdomen, torso, and extremity surgery.

If one wishes to create from the standpoint of medical history the category of a "medical first" in the field of aesthetic plastic surgery, without becoming too overly involved in the problem of historic semantics, we can probably trace the concept of aesthetic plastic surgery to J. F. Dieffenbach (1792–1847) (Fig. 1). Many considered Dieffenbach the most skillful plastic surgeon in the mid-nineteenth century, and his reputation was so great that when he visited Paris all the hospitals were made available to him for his surgery (8, 31). For narrowing thick nostril walls, for example, Dieffenbach advised cutting out small

---

Address reprint requests to Blair O. Rogers, M.D., 875 Fifth Avenue, New York, N.Y. 10021.

1

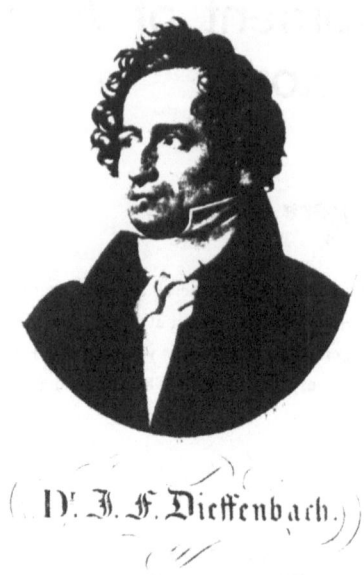

D! J. F. Dieffenbach.

Fig. 1. Johann Friedrich Dieffenbach (1792–1847). (Courtesy of Dr. V. J. Bernbeck.)

punched-shaped pieces of skin and cartilage, reducing their thickness by tension of the skin closure (Fig. 2). He also removed externally a vertical and horizontal piece of skin and subcutaneous tissue bilaterally, with the skin closure reducing the size of an overly large nose (Fig. 3). His method of raising a flattened or depressed nasal tip through an external incisional approach is seen in Figure 4.

The use of external incisions for any and all nasal corrective (aesthetic) or reconstructive surgery was routine in the mid-nineteenth century, and any thought of an intranasal approach seems to have escaped the surgeons of that era and did not have its origins until the paper of Roe (54) in 1887. The history of corrective (aesthetic) surgery cannot, however, be divorced from the history of reconstructive plastic surgery. Even today one is reminded daily how interwoven these two types of surgery are and always have been. A quote from Gillies' and Millard's classic textbook (13) is appropriate here:

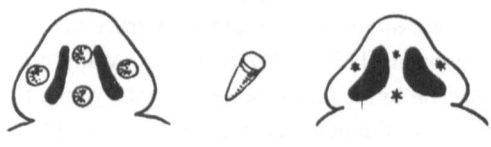

DIEFFENBACH METHOD.

Fig. 2. Dieffenbach's method of narrowing thick nostril walls by the excision of small punched-shaped pieces of skin and cartilage. (From ref. 28, p. 467.)

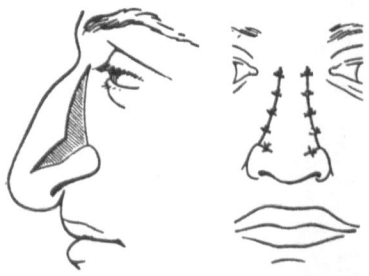 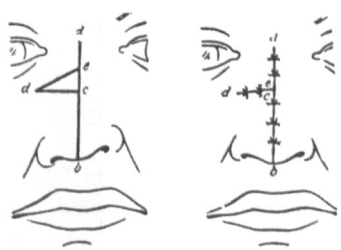

Fig. 3. Dieffenbach's method of using external excisions to reduce the size of an overly large, hooked, drooping nose. (From ref. 7, p. 484.)

Fig. 4. Dieffenbach's method of using external excisions to raise a flattened or depressed nasal tip. (From ref. 7, p. 483.)

A great percentage of private practice is beauty surgery. It is here that perfection is a necessity. Reconstructive surgery is an attempt to return to normal; cosmetic surgery is an attempt to surpass the normal. No man is a plastic surgeon unless he becomes adept at both. Many never do and are a menace. It is easier to reduce than produce, but in plastic surgery it is nearly always necessary to remould after reduction. Thus anyone can cut off a bit of a nose or breast, but not so many can turn out a satisfying result. (13)

Unless it can be proven otherwise by more definitive and accurate translations of Dieffenbach's articles dealing with ear reconstruction (8), the first true correction of a protruding ear was performed in 1881 by Ely (10), a young otolaryngologic surgeon. The patient on whom he operated and reported his surgery in the Manhattan Eye, Ear and Throat Hospital Annual Report can be seen in Figure 5. Ely had a short life and died at the age of 37 from tuberculosis caused by his extreme dedication and exhaustive overwork.

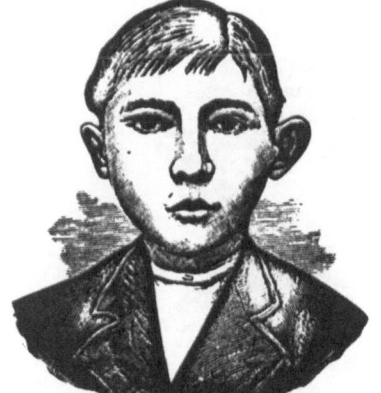 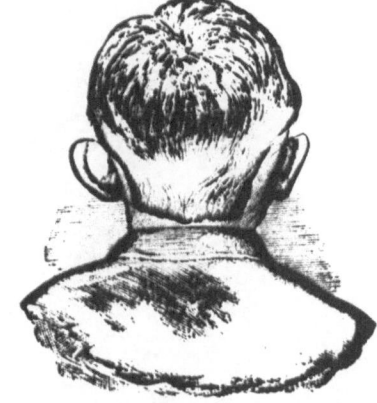

Fig. 5. Preoperative and postoperative illustration of the first patient operated on by Ely in 1881 for correction of protruding ears. (From Ely, E. T.: Plast. Reconstr. Surg. 42:583, 1968.)

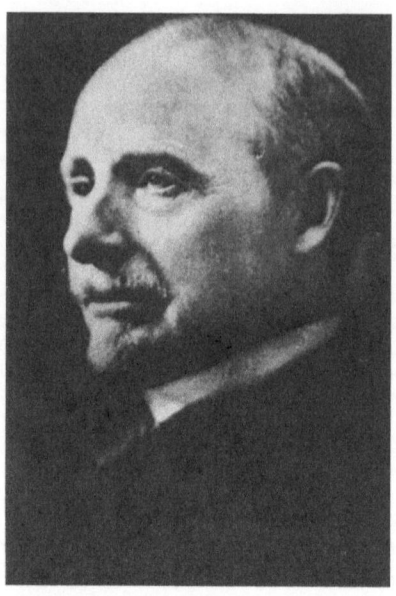

Fig. 6. John Orlando Roe, father of aesthetic rhinoplasty (1848–1915). (From Cottle, M. H.: Arch. Otolaryngol. 80:22, 1964.

The age of corrective aesthetic rhinoplasty began in 1887, when John Orlando Roe (1848–1915), an otolaryngologist from Rochester, New York (Fig. 6), described an intranasal operation confined to the tip of a so-called pug nose. With the title of "The Deformity termed Pug Nose and Its Correction by a Simple Operation" (54), he described in his article an intranasal operation confined to the tip of the nose (Fig. 7). His publication in 1891 of another paper, "The Correction of Angular Deformities of the Nose by a Sub-

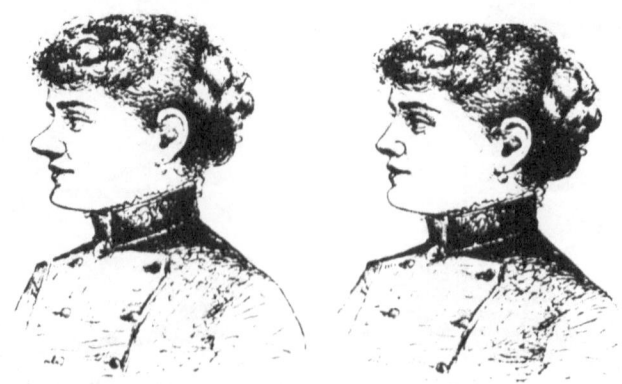

Fig. 7. Illustration of patient pre- and postoperatively in Roe's first article in 1887 for correction of a "pug nose." (From ref. 54)

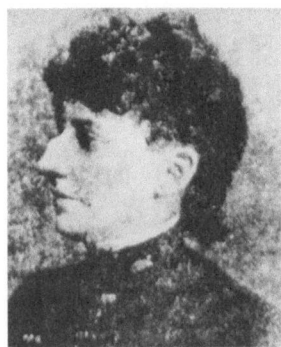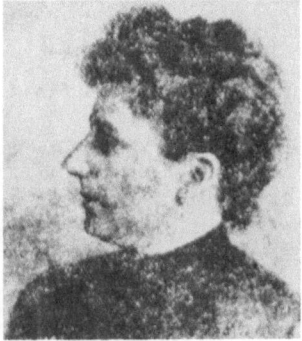

Fig. 8. First photographic illustration of pre- and postoperative condition of patient with correction of an entire nasal deformity in Roe's second paper, in 1891. (From ref. 55.)

cutaneous Operation" (55), was more truly the medical first, since it described corrective rhinoplasty of the entire nose in which the nose was reduced in size throughout because of a prominent bony and cartilaginous hump and profile (Fig. 8).

A more detailed chronologic survey of the development of aesthetic and corrective rhinoplasty just before the age of Roe and immediately after the introduction of his contributions is given by Rogers in a recently published article in an international symposium on aesthetic plastic surgery of the nose titled "Early Historical Rhinoplasty" (61).

Roe's second paper in 1891 reporting his intranasal subcutaneous approach to aesthetic rhinoplasty was written 7 years before Jacques Joseph reported similar success using external incisions (1, 19). Roe performed his operations under local cocaine anesthesia. He undermined the skin widely, inserted an angulated bone scissors, and cut off the hump until the dorsum was smooth. At the end of the operation he strapped the skin down with external pressure and a splint. There is no doubt on the part of medical historians today

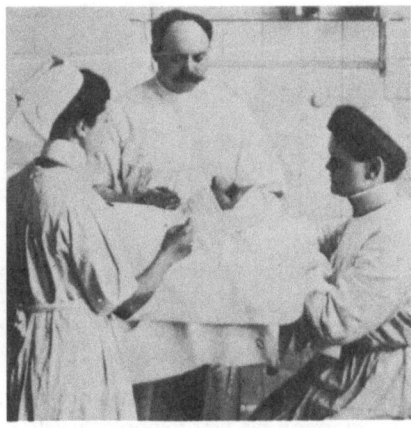

Fig. 9. Jacques Joseph with nurse assistants. (From ref. 26.)

5

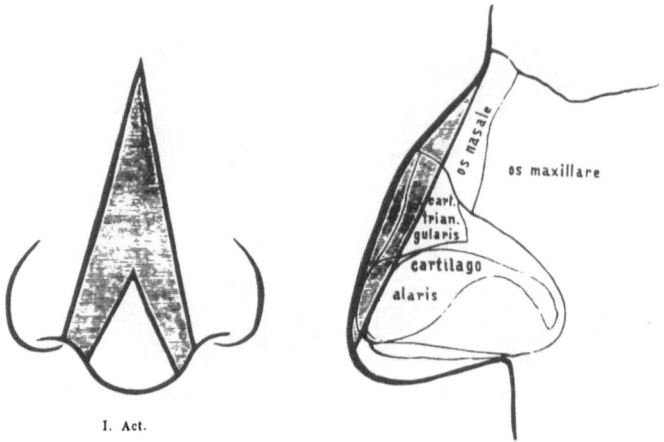

Fig. 10. First illustration by Jacques Joseph of the use of external excisions to reduce the size of an overly conspicuous nose. (From ref. 19.)

that these two papers of 1887 and 1891 established Roe as the originator of corrective or cosmetic rhinoplasty, despite Joseph's claim to this title. In all fairness to Joseph, however, who came on the scene in 1898, no one disagrees (because of Joseph's accomplishments) with modern historians who call him the overall father of corrective aesthetic rhinoplasty.

In 1898 Jacques Joseph of Berlin (Fig. 9), whose life is indeed fascinating (47), excised externally an inverted V-shaped segment along the nasal dorsum through the skin, bone, cartilage, and mucosal lining, and the entire thickness of the nasal alae, and removed a wedge from the lower part of the septum to shorten and reduce an overly conspicuous nose all in one single operation (Fig. 10). Figure 11 shows the preoperative and postoperative

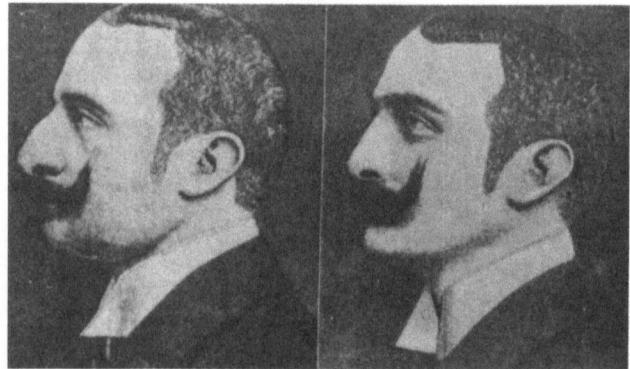

Fig. 11. Pre- and postoperative photographs of the "28-year-old landowner" on whom Joseph performed his first rhinoplasty with external excisions. (From ref. 19.)

photographs of the "28-year-old (male) landowner" on whom Joseph performed this operation.

He published a second paper (20) in 1902, noting that he had then performed 10 such cosmetic operations but was still using external skin incisions and excisions through which he removed the hump and shortened the nose. By 1904, while Roe reported continued successes in America using intranasal incisions, Joseph (22) admitted that he had finally come around to using intranasal incisions instead of his previously employed external skin incisions, and by that year he had performed 43 operations. In another paper (21) in 1904, Joseph described for the first time his external clamps and his right-angle nasal saws, and by 1905 he reported (23) that he had operated on 100 patients requiring corrective rhinoplasty. In another paper, in 1905, he emphasized the use of plaster casts and carefully taken photographs for studying each patient and the value of these items in assessing postoperative results.

Although numerous papers describing reconstructive ophthalmic plastic surgery were written from the time of von Graefe (58) in 1818 and onward, especially papers describing excess skin folds of the eyelids first published by Mackenzie in 1830 and others who advised excision of the excess skin alone, the true aesthetic surgery of baggy or excessively wrinkled eyelids did not develop until the early 1900s. The earliest attempts to remove excess skin only can be traced to Charles Conrad Miller (59, 60) who, in 1906, wrote his first exclusively aesthetic surgery article on the excision of "bag-like folds of eyelid skin" (33). One year later in another article there appeared probably the first photograph in medical history illustrating the lower eyelid incisions required for removal of a crescent of wrinkled skin (Fig. 12) (39). Miller's career in cosmetic surgery, as he preferred to call it, was, therefore, already well underway (32–41, 59, 60). Unfortunately, this tragic man was both a quack and a surgical visionary, years ahead of his more academic colleagues. He lived and practiced in Chicago, the epicenter of North American folklore, folk songs, folk poetry, folk nostrums, and folk medicines. Is it any wonder, then, that medicine's first truly cosmetic surgeon, Charles Conrad Miller, hung his shingle at 100 State Street in Chicago in 1903, having just graduated from the Hospital College of Medicine of Louisville, Kentucky in 1902? Perhaps a gift of gab or a "confidence-man" personality and, even more importantly, his gift for writing voluminously in the medical literature brought to his office what we assume were hundreds of men and women seeking youth and attractiveness.

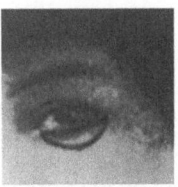

Fig. 12. The line of incision for removal of a crescent of skin to correct excess "bagging," folding, or wrinkling of the eyelid skin. (From ref. 39.)

7

The Correction

OF

Featural Imperfections

BY

CHARLES C. MILLER, M. D.

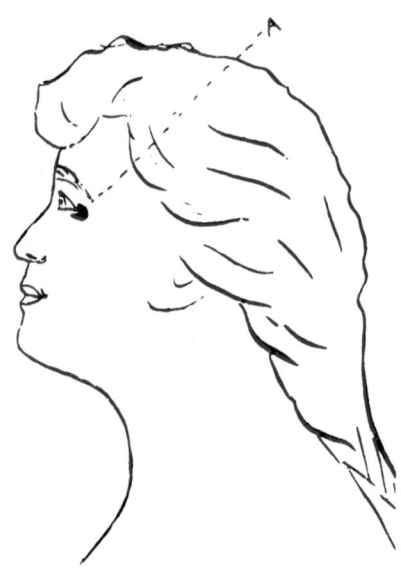

PUBLISHED BY THE AUTHOR
70 STATE ST., CHICAGO

Oak Printing Co., 9 Wendell St.

Fig. 13. Title page of C. C. Miller's first book on cosmetic surgery, published in 1907. (From ref. 35.)

Fig. 14. Area to be excised for correction of crow's feet. (From ref. 41.)

It is obvious from reading Miller's paper on eyelid surgery, written in 1906, that his career in aesthetic surgery had already been well underway for several years before that article. In 1907 Miller published the first book in medical history (35) written on cosmetic surgery (Fig. 13), and a second, slightly enlarged edition appeared in 1908 (41). From 1907 onward, Miller contributed to the literature a host of other articles on cosmetic surgery subjects. He had already shown interest in cosmetic correction of the hump nose (32) in 1906, in correction of crow's feet in 1907 (40) (Fig. 14), and can be assumed to have experimented with paraffin injections for several years before the publication of a book on this subject in 1908 (44).

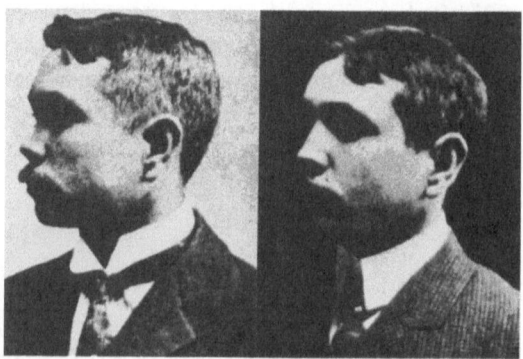

Fig. 15. Photographs preoperatively and post-paraffin injection to correct a nasal deformity. (From Annual Reports of Manhattan Eye, Ear and Throat Hospital, 1904.)

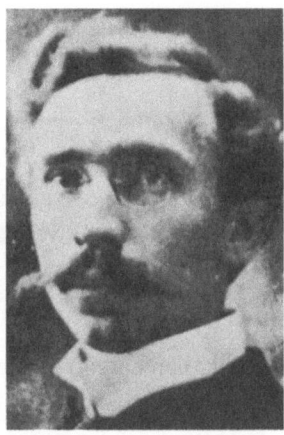

Fig. 16. Portrait of the German-born American cosmetic surgeon, Frederick Strange Kolle. (From Grigg, E. R. N.: The Trail of the Invisible Light. Charles C Thomas, Springfield, Ill., 1965.)

Several years before Miller's first surgical paper was published, injections of vaseline for the correction of facial defects were described by Gersuny (12). Vaseline injections were soon discarded because of unfavorable results and especially because of complications including severe local tissue reactions and distant emboli, with some cases of fatal pulmonary emboli. In 1902 Eckstein described the injection of low-melting paraffin (9). For approximately the next 20 years or more, many physicians unfortunately injected paraffin with immediately good results, as seen in Figure 15, which shows a patient injected for the treatment of a nasal deformity by a surgeon on the staff of the Manhattan Eye, Ear and Throat Hospital in 1904. Paraffin injections were finally discarded after many years of trial however, because of local paraffinoma formation and distant complications, which included thrombosis, phlebitis, pulmonary emboli, and infarction. These injections of vaseline and paraffin in the first two decades of the twentieth century served as one of the major drawbacks of this era, delaying the more rapid and accepted development of corrective cosmetic surgery in general, and corrective nasoplastic surgery in particular, because all too frequently good cosmetic surgeons such as Frederick Strange Kolle (1871–1929) also were susceptible to the blandishments of quick results obtainable through paraffin injections (27).

Chronologically, the second author in medical history to describe cosmetic surgery was Kolle (Fig. 16), a German-born American who practiced plastic and cosmetic surgery in New York City. In 1911 Kolle published a book entitled *Plastic and Cosmetic Surgery* (28). This large tome consisted of 511 pages and 522 illustrations, among which were some of the first photographs of a patient before and after the surgical correction of protruding ears (Fig. 17). Kolle's most interesting contribution was his treatment of wrinkled eyelids; he included illustrations (Fig. 18) that described his methods of correction. Miller's operation on the eyelids was less refined, but both men attacked the problem from

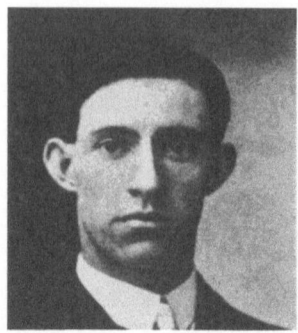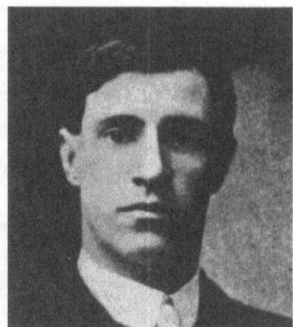

Fig. 17. Correction of protruding ears: pre- and postoperative photographs. (From ref. 28, p. 142.)

approximately the same primitive standpoint. In his book Kolle stated that massage accomplished little in the correction of wrinkled eyelids. It should be noted that Kolle was quite bold, for he removed eyelid sutures as early as 24 to 48 hours after the operation. Because of the edema that usually followed operations on the eyelids during this pre-antibiotic era, Kolle advised that the upper and lower lids be treated in separate operations.

In 1912, one year after the publication of Kolle's book, Eugen Holländer (1867–1932) of Berlin, a pupil of the famous James Israel, stated in a chapter entitled "Cosmetic Surgery" that at one time "as a victim of the art of feminine persuasion," he removed pieces of skin at the margins of the hairline and in the natural aging skin folds of a woman to "freshen up" her wrinkles and drooping cheeks (15). He did not state in this chapter the year in which he performed this operation, nor did he illustrate or describe any further surgical details of this single operation. After 1912 he devoted himself largely to writing several outstanding books that dealt primarily with medicine and surgery as depicted in paintings, illustrations, caricatures, and satire in the entire historic period from the art of Ancient Greece up to his time. One of Holländer's most famous books, *Medicine in Classical Paintings,* was first published in 1903 (14).

In the year of his death in 1932, probably aware of the increasing number of articles appearing in the surgical literature dealing with facelifting techniques, and using obvious surgical hindsight, Holländer wrote that it was actually in 1901 that he was sought by a Polish aristocrat who wished to have a facelift performed (16). Until 1901, according to

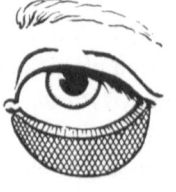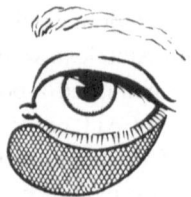

Fig. 18. Shape of incisions in lower eyelids for removal of loose tissue causing eyelid wrinkles. (From ref. 28, p. 116.)

10

Holländer, this operation was completely unknown. The woman had made a drawing that essentially demonstrated to him that through the removal of facial skin taken up in front of the ear, a favorable adjustment of the nasolabial folds and an elevation of the corners of the mouth would occur. At first he resisted the idea of performing the operation, especially because this probably would have been the first time that such a surgical feat had been attempted (16). But because of "feminine persuasion" he did carry it out, apparently with success (15). In the early stages of developing his surgical technique, Holländer excised only isolated "pieces of skin" in the hair region or at the border of the hair, and behind the ear, but his results in these early cases were "inferior" (16). His early operation had little effect on wrinkles in the lower portions of the face.

The next surgeon on the scene, who similarly relied on surgical hindsight many years later, was Erich Lexer (1867–1937). In 1931 Lexer stated that he had not heard of any previous surgical attempts at facelifting when he performed such an operation on an actress in 1906. Before seeking him out, she customarily put her facial skin under tension at night by drawing up on it with pieces of sticking plaster held under tension by strips of rubber pulled over the vault of her skull. Long-standing use of this apparatus had caused pronounced transverse tension folds above her zygomatic arches, and she wanted these folds removed surgically. Lexer stated in his typical fashion, "a single attempt (at this surgery) was successful!" (29).

In Lexer's facelift operation, as he described it in 1931, S-shaped incisions of skin were made in the temporal region in front of and behind the ear, and elliptical excisions were made in the forehead or frontal region. The incisions at the lower border of the ear began at the insertion of the lobule in the preauricular region (Fig. 19). After excising the redun-

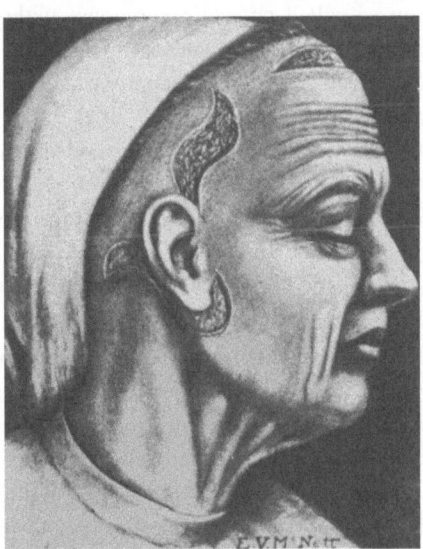

Fig. 19. Artist's adaptation of Fig. 1290 in Lexer (Die gesamte Wiederherstellungschirurgie. Leipzig, Barth, 1931). (From May, H.: Reconstructive and Reparative Surgery. F.A. Davis, Philadelphia, 1947, p. 146.)

11

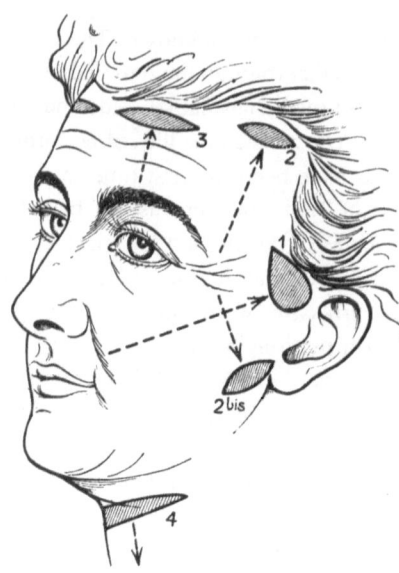

Fig. 20. Different types of small skin excisions necessary for correction of facial wrinkles. (From ref. 50.)

dant skin, Lexer anchored the subcutaneous sutures behind the ear to the periosteum of the mastoid region. Lexer stated that it was clear to them from the very beginning that because of the elasticity of the facial skin, a mere simple closure of small skin excisions performed in his day by many so-called cosmetic surgeons, without undermining of the wound defects, resulted in only a short-lived success. Therefore, he decided even in his first case in 1906 not to be content with a simple approximation of the wound edges, but through the use of deep sutures to anchor the edges of the skin flaps to the temporalis fascia. The cutting off of little "spindles" of skin, he said derisively, had little or only short-lived success. This same reason can undoubtedly apply to many of the so-called minilifts of today, no matter what exaggerated claims are made for them by their so-called inventors.

With the end of the First World War in 1918, surgeons who probably had an interest in plastic surgery before or at the beginning of the war, and who had put their interests aside because of the wartime need for their reconstructive surgical services, began publishing articles that had probably been unwritten during the war years. The most important of these—the first article that illustrated fully the multiple small elliptical or ovoid excisions of skin, which were then being employed (similar to the minilifts of today)—appeared in the May 12, 1919 issue of *La Presse Médicale*. It was written by Raymond Passot (1886–1933) (50), a pupil of Hippolyte Morestin. In order to obtain an upward and/or lateral suspensory tension on various facial wrinkles, Passot excised small pieces of skin in separate areas of the forehead at the scalp hairline, or adjacent to the pretemporal areas, and in the preauricular region adjacent to the attachment of the ear lobule (Fig. 20).

In addition, the diagram included in Passot's first 1919 article demonstrates that he was also concerned with the "double chin" problem, and perhaps he was the first in the literature to describe an attempt at its correction by the removal of a long ellipse of skin either next to or just below the hyoid, together with its underlying fatty tissue (50). All skin defects created by these multiple excisions were drawn together under tension with horsehair sutures, still in common use at the end of the war. Passot felt that the best postoperative results, which lasted for many years, were obtained in relatively younger women in whom the skin had not "totally collapsed." He was perhaps the first to mention in the literature the stimulating effect and the serious social value these operations had on the morale of the person operated on (51).

Passot reminded his readers that reparative (reconstructive) surgery went through its period of suspicion and skepticism on the part of the medical profession before the war, and that cosmetic surgery soon after the war was probably undergoing a similar experience, which would subside within several years. It was only through numerous publications and trials that the good results of major reconstructive plastic surgical operations proved themselves worthwhile to the medical profession at large. The "prodigious" rise of reconstructive surgery of the face during World War I erased the last bits of skepticism in the medical community. Passot remembered hearing Morestin say that a majority of patients who suffered facial mutilation before the war preferred wearing a prosthesis to submitting to a total plastic surgical reconstruction. Passot colorfully wrote that if reconstructive surgery in 1919 had, by its proven wartime ability, literally received "keys of the city," it might also be said that cosmetic surgery purely and simply still remained "in quarantine."

One month after the publication of Passot's pioneering article (50), at the annual meeting of the Alumni Association of The University of Oregon's Medical School in Portland in late June 1919, Dr. Adalbert G. Bettman (1883–1964) of the same city was probably the first in medical literature to demonstrate to his audience before and after photographs

Fig. 21. Pre- and postoperative views. First photographic illustrations (1920) in medical literature of the results of a facelift operation. (From ref. 2.)

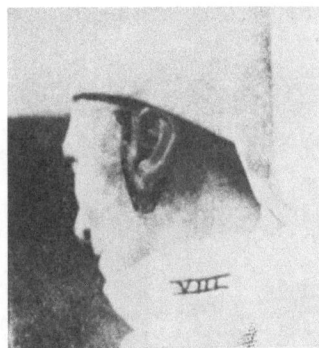

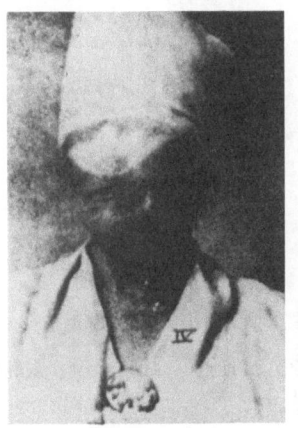
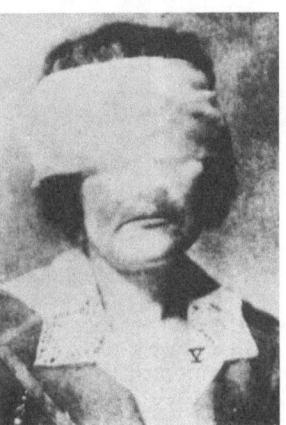

Fig. 22. First photographic illustration (1920) of complete preauricular and posterior auricular incision employed for the facelift operation as we know it today. (From ref. 2.)

of a facelift operation. These photographs were subsequently published in an article in *Northwest Medicine* in August 1920 (Figs. 21 and 22) (2). Although Bettman spoke of removing from the temporal and preauricular regions small pieces of skin varying in size from the size of a dime to that of a half dollar, Figure VIII in his 1920 article (Fig. 22) showed for the "first time" in medical history a very extensive incision extending up into the temporal region, down along the preauricular region, and under and behind the ear lobule. This is essentially the same preauricular and posterior auricular incision as is used today in the many modified versions in both shape and extent of what we now call the typical facelift operation. Thus, for all intents and purposes, in assigning medical firsts from the standpoint of actual publication in the literature, we should treat Bettman as the "father" of the total facelift operation.

Five months after Passot's first article in May 1919, Julien Bourguet of Paris similarly described the use of small, crescent-shaped, angular or *gendarme-hat*-shaped incisions to correct forehead wrinkles, crow's feet, and neck wrinkles, respectively. These descriptions were published in October 1919, but the drawings illustrating Bourguet's technique, which were part of his Academy of Medicine lecture, were not included in the published version of his paper. Considering the morale and the psychologic suffering of persons with wrinkles, Bourguet was perhaps one of the first to emphasize that although men with nasal deformities suffer as much as women because of the aesthetics of an unpleasant nose, they are indifferent to or much less concerned with facial wrinkles than women are. He believed that the skin of men usually remained more firm and more well-preserved with aging than the skin of women (4).

Five years later, in November 1924, Bourguet was probably the first to describe his technique for the excisional correction of pockets of herniated peri-orbital fat (bags) of the eyelid region (5); and in 1925 he also probably was the first in medical history to publish before and after photographs of patients (6) who had undergone this cosmetic blepharoplastic operation (Fig. 23) as well as the double chin corrective procedure (Fig. 24). Rather than incising the eyelid skin, Bourguet approached these fat herniations through

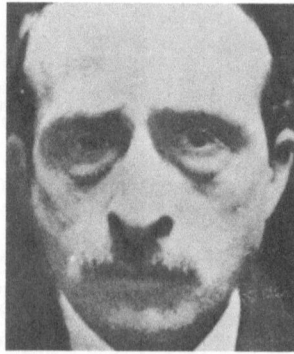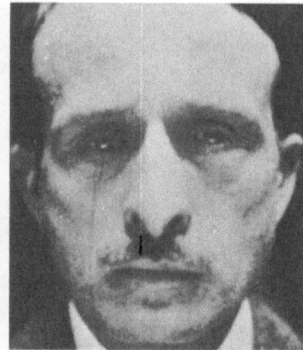

Fig. 23. First photograph in medical literature (1925) of before and after results of removing "bags" in the lower eyelids. (From ref. 6.)

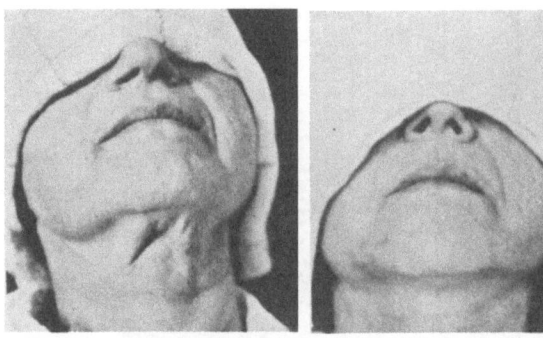

Fig. 24. First photographs in medical literature (1925) of before and after results in correction of the double chin. (From ref. 6.)

the mucosa of the conjunctival cul-de-sac of the lower eyelid (5, 6). Several catgut sutures were used to close the fibrous sac or capsule, which usually surrounds the fatty herniated masses.

Despite the innumerable small incisions Charles Conrad Miller recommended (46) to be made in the eyelid skin, as illustrated and described in his expanded 1925 book on cosmetic surgery, Miller never included any before and after photographs in his book, nor did he mention the role of peri-orbital fat herniation as one of the glaring deformities in many patients who complain of "aging eyelids."

Jacques Joseph (1865–1934) of Berlin also used surgical hindsight in 1921, reminding his readers that he too had performed an operation as far back as 1912 for correction of the redundant aging cheek tissues of a 48-year-old woman (24). Thus a series of events, recalled only with surgical hindsight by their authors, has been passed down in the medical literature. These events in the gradual development of facelifting as a surgical procedure are attributable to three men: Holländer (1901), Lexer (1906), and Joseph (1912). Each of these German surgeons told his readers years *after the fact* that he had performed the facelifting operation many years and even decades previously (15, 16, 29, 24). But to be truly fair, from the standpoint of medical history, it should be emphasized that from their actual date of publication, some of the earliest descriptions in the literature for the surgical correction of isolated areas of facial wrinkling must, without doubt, be credited first to Miller (33, 35, 36–43) from 1906 to 1909, and secondly to Kolle (28) in 1911, both of them Americans.

To Joseph in 1921, however, belongs the credit of being the second surgeon after Bettman (2) to publish before and after photographs of the results of a facelift operation (Fig. 25). In truth, his photographic results seem to be superior to Bettman's, and surprisingly enough, Bettman's actual incision, described a year earlier, seems to be almost identical to that described in Joseph's 1921 article. Joseph was perhaps the first to emphasize (24) the sociologic aspects in cosmetic surgery to which those few men who published before him had not drawn attention. He referred specifically to the early appearance of aging wrinkles in women between the ages of 40 and 50, wrinkles which quite frequently

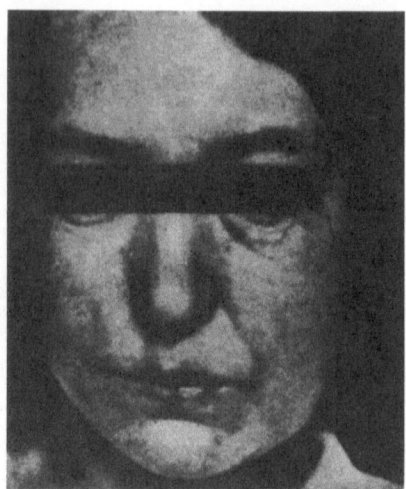

Fig. 25. Right side of patient's face has already been corrected by a facelift procedure; left side is as yet uncorrected, showing advantages of the "lifting" operation. (From ref. 24.)

could interfere with their earning a living if they were working women. This was a rather refreshing change in the literature in contrast to other writers who referred only to Polish aristocrats and famous actresses. In September 1912 Joseph's first patient, a 48-year-old woman, gave a history of seeking a position in business but being unable to obtain it because of her prematurely aged appearance.

In 1922, again in *Northwest Medicine,* another American, F. A. Booth of Seattle, Washington, published his technique for correcting facial sagging with the use of a facelift incision essentially similar to that described by Joseph and by Bettman several years earlier (3). Interestingly, Booth also presented a new variation, quite practical, for correcting the double chin (Fig. 26).

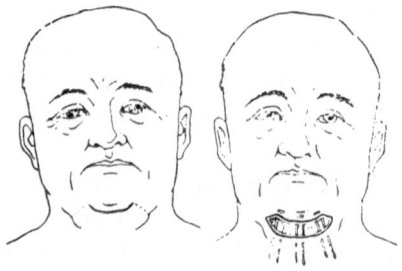

Fig. 26. Curved line incision under the chin for removal of double chin; dotted area demonstrates amount of dissection and undermining necessary for removal of excessive fat. Right: The amount of excised submental skin, with retention mattress sutures inserted to obliterate the "dead space," thus correcting the double chin. (From ref. 3.)

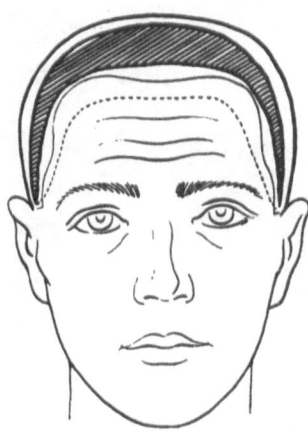

Fig. 27. An incision behind the hairline extending from one temporal region to the other, with hair-bearing skin as much as 0.5 to 0.75 in. wide at the midline excised to correct horizontal frown lines (a procedure largely abandoned by most surgeons today). (From ref. 18.)

Another fascinating man in the early history of American cosmetic surgery was Harold Napier Lyons Hunt (1882–1954) of New York City (18). In 1926, the same year that Madame Noël's famous book appeared (48), Hunt's book *Plastic Surgery of the Head, Face and Neck* was published (18). In it Hunt described not only facelifting operations, but forehead or brow lifting operations (Fig. 27), as well as procedures for correcting a double chin. He was another prolific writer whose interests ranged beyond plastic surgery, and actually after 1926 Hunt's interests in the latter field declined considerably because he devoted himself chiefly to treating impotence by the transplantation of ram and sheep glands (17).

In closing this brief review of the early development of aesthetic or cosmetic surgery of the facial region, it is almost mandatory to refer to one of the most remarkable people and the first woman in the history of aesthetic surgery. An early pioneer in the development of facelifting and eyelid plasty techniques was Madame le Dr. A. (Suzanne) Noël (Fig. 28) (52), whose book *La Chirurgie Esthétique: Son Rôle Social* appeared in 1926 (48). A German translation of this book appeared 6 years later (49). Chronologically, hers was the sixth medical book devoted almost solely to cosmetic surgery published in the early twentieth century, after those of Miller (35, 41, 46), Kolle (28), and Hunt (18).

Noël stated that her interest in cosmetic surgery began in 1912 when one of the great actresses of France returned from America after a triumphant tour (48, 52, 59, 60). All of the newspapers remarked how, by means of a practical operation on the scalp, she had regained a surprising youthfulness. Thus some type of facelifting procedure was already being performed in America before or at least during 1912 by a surgeon or surgeons not identified by name. Impressed by these newspaper reports, Noël pinched the skin of her

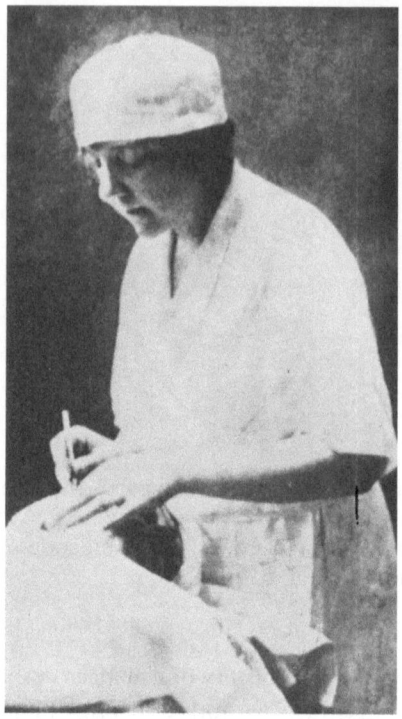

Fig. 28. Dr. Suzanne Noël, the world's first female cosmetic plastic surgeon, (From ref. 53, p. 461.)

own face with her fingers in different places and in different directions to try to adjust the skin folds. She was surprised by what she was able to accomplish merely by lifting her facial skin with her fingers so she began to study this question seriously. Noël devised wooden clips, experimented with them in living anesthetized rabbits, and found that when

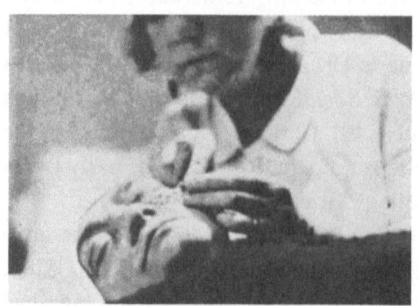
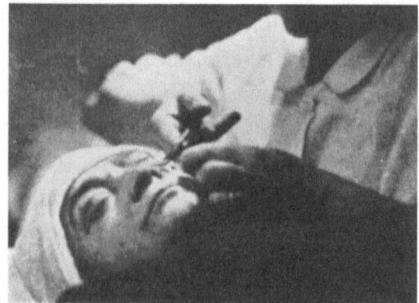

Fig. 29. Dr. Noël operating on a female patient for "bags" of the eyelids. Note the absence of any facial mask or surgical gloves. (From ref. 48.)

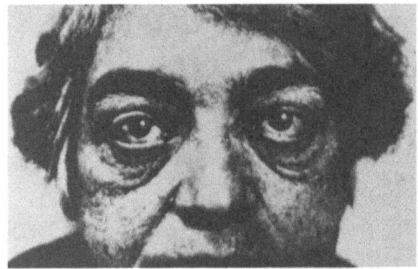
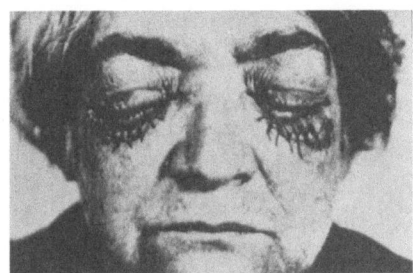
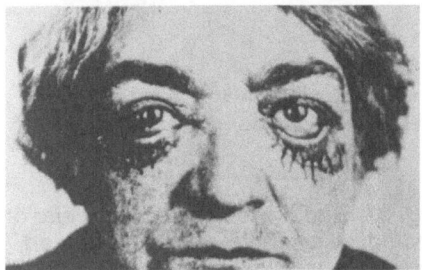
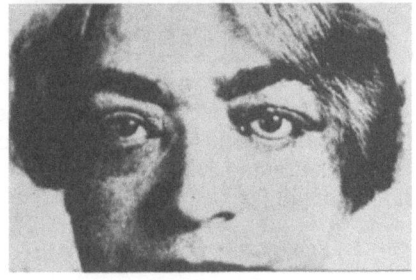

Fig. 30. Top: One of Dr. Noël's patients before excision of "bags" and wrinkles of lower eyelid skin. Bottom: Patient immediately postoperative with operative sutures in place, eyes open. (From ref. 48.)

Fig. 31. Same patient as in Fig. 30. Top: operative sutures in place with eyes closed. Bottom: Results 15 days postoperatively. (From ref. 48.)

applied to the skin the clips produced the same "lifting results" as she previously achieved with her fingers.

It was probably during World War I, and not until 1916, that Noël first met the famous surgeon de Martel, one of Passot's teachers, and sought his advice on her projects and the means by which she was hoping to solve the facelifting problem. As with Passot, de Martel influenced Noël considerably and she was deeply grateful. Her cosmetic surgery book was the only one of the five previously mentioned that included numerous photographs—59 pre- and postoperative photographs of the results of her skillful surgery. Among those subjects described in detail in a book containing 11 operative illustrations and 51 photographs of technique for surgical correction are baggy eyelids (Figs. 29 through 31); facial (Figs. 32 and 33), forehead, eyelid, and neck wrinkles; and double chins. Also discussed are correction of redundant neck skin by massive excision of skin and scalp tissue in the nape of the neck and in the suboccipital scalp region; the excision of large nevi (hairy and otherwise) of the breast, neck, and posterior auricular regions; the correction of keloidal burn scars of the neck, of flabby tissues of the arms of aging women, and of protruding ears; and the excision of forearm tattoos. As one can see from perus-

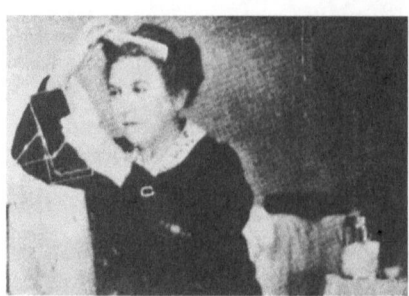

Fig. 32. Middle-aged patient combs her hair preparing to go home after a temporal facelift performed in Dr. Noël's office. (From ref. 48.)

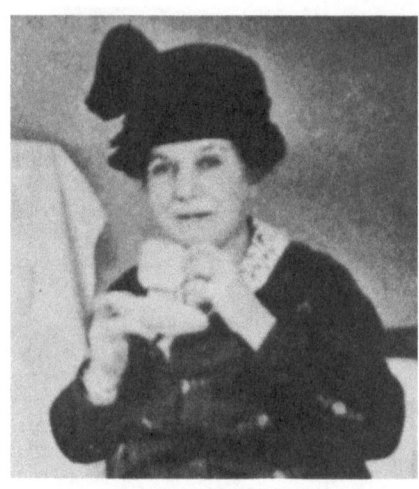

Fig. 33. Middle-aged patient at the end of a temporal facelift operation performed under local anesthesia in Dr. Noël's office. (From ref. 48.)

ing her text, Noël was a very versatile surgeon. Moreover, she wrote in a charming, warm, and thoroughly womanly fashion, as attested to in the fascinating article written about her recently by Paule Regnault (52), one of her pupils.

It might be fitting at the close of this brief historic review to consider the gentle smile on the face of a patient who has just undergone a facelift operation performed under local anesthesia in Dr. Noël's office. The patient has put her handsome bonnet on, is ready to go home, and is calmly drinking a cup of coffee (Figs. 32 and 33). Perhaps her happy, confident, and pleased expression is symbolic of the attitude of most patients who, since those early years of our specialty more than half a century ago, have undergone aesthetic plastic surgery with all of the postoperative, physical, psychologic, and social improvements that are the most rewarding aspects of this most delightful and satisfying branch of the overall practice of plastic and reconstructive surgery.

References

1. Aufricht, G.: Commentary on the paper: operative reduction on the size of a nose (rhinomyosis) by Jacques Joseph. Plast. Reconstr. Surg. 46:181, 1970.
2. Bettman, A. G.: Plastic and cosmetic surgery of the face. Northwest Med. 19:205, 1920.
3. Booth F. A.: Cosmetic surgery of the face, neck and breast. Northwest Med. 21:170, 1922.
4. Bourguet, J.: II: La disparition chirurgicale des rides et plis du visage. Bull. Acad. Méd. (Paris) 82:183, 1919
5. Bourguet, J.: V. Les hernies graisseuses de l'orbite. Notre traitement chirurgical. Bull. Acad. Méd. (Paris), 92:1270, 1924.
6. Bourguet, J.: Chirurgie esthétique de la face: Les nez concaves, les rides et les "poches" sous les yeux. Arch. Prov. Chir. 28:293, 1925.

7. Davis, J. S.: Plastic Surgery: Its Principles and Practice. P. Blakiston's, Philadelphia, 1919.

8. Dieffenbach, J. F.: Die operative Chirurgie. F. A. Brockhaus, Leipzig, 1845.

9. Eckstein, H.: Ueber subkutane und submukose Hartparaffinprothesen. Dtsch. Med. Wochenschr. 28:573, 1902.

10. Ely, E. T.: An operation for prominence of the auricles. Arch. Otolaryngol. 10:97, 1881; also in Plast. Reconstr. Surg., 42:582, 1968.

11. Garrison, F. H.: An Introduction to the History of Medicine, 4th ed. W. B. Saunders, Philadelphia, 1929, pp. 29, 494.

12. Gersuny, R.: Ueber eine subcutane Prothese. Z. Heilkd. 1:199, 1900.

13. Gillies, H. D., and Millard, D. R., Jr.: The Principles and Art of Plastic Surgery. Little, Brown & Co., Boston, 1957.

14. Holländer, E.: Die Medizin in der klassischen Malerei. F. Enke, Stuttgart, 1903.

15. Holländer, E.: XVII. Die kosmetische Chirurgie. In Joseph, M. (ed.): Handbuch der Kosmetik. Verlag von Veit, Leipzig, 1912, p. 688.

16. Holländer, E.: Plastische (Kosmetische) Operation: Kritische Darstellung ihres gegenwärtigen Standes. In Klemperer, G. and Klemperer, F. (eds.): Neue Deutsche Klinik, vol. 9. Urban and Schwarzenberg, Berlin, 1932, pp. 1–17.

17. Hunt, H. L.: New theory of the function of the prostate deduced from gland transplantation in physicians. Endocrinology 9:479, 1925.

18. Hunt, H. L.: Plastic Surgery of the Head, Face and Neck. Lea & Febiger, Philadelphia, 1926.

19. Joseph, J.: Über die operative Verkleinerung einer Nase (Rhinomiosis) Berl. Klin. Wochenschr. 40:882, 1898.

20. Joseph, J.: Ueber einige weitere Nasenverkleinerungen. Berl. Klin. Wochenschr. p. 851, 1902.

21. Joseph, J.: Nasenverkleinerungen. Deutsch. Med. Wochenschr. 30:1095, 1904.

22. Joseph, J.: Intranasale Nasenhöckerabtragung. Berl. Klin. Wochenschr. p. 650, 1904.

23. Joseph, J.: Weiteres über Nasenverkleinerungen. Münch. Med. Wochenschr. 52:1489, 1905.

24. Joseph, J.: Hängewangenplastik(Melomioplastik). Dtsch. Med. Wochenschr. 47:287, 1921.

25. Joseph, J.: Verbesserung meiner Hängewangenplastik (Melomioplastik). Dtsch. Med. Wochenschr. 54:567, 1928.

26. Joseph, J.: Nasenplastik und sonstige Gesichtsplastik nebst einem Anhang über Mammaplastik. Verlag von Curt Kabitzsch, Leipzig, 1928–1931.

27. Kolle, F. S.: Subcutaneous Hydrocarbon Prostheses. The Grafton Press, New York, 1908.

28. Kolle, F. S.: Plastic and Cosmetic Surgery. D. Appleton and Co., New York, 1911.

29. Lexer, E.: Die gesamte Wiederherstellungschirurgie, vol. 2. J. A. Barth, Leipzig, 1931, p. 548.

30. May, H.: Erich Lexer: A biographical sketch. Plast. Reconstr. Surg. 29:141, 1962.

31. McDowell, F., Vallone, J. A., and Brown, J. B.: Bibliography and historical note on plastic surgery of the nose. Plast. Reconstr. Surg. 10:149, 1952.

32. Miller, C. C.: Surgical treatment of hump nose. Med. Brief 34:160, 1906.

33. Miller, C. C.: The excision of bag-like folds of skin from the region about the eyes. Med. Brief 34:648, 1906.

34. Miller, C. C.: The surgical reduction of the nasal tip of excessive length. Ala. Med. J. 19:620, 1906.

35. Miller, C. C.: The Correction of Featural Imperfections. Oak Printing Co., Chicago, 1907.

36. Miller, C. C.: Semilunar excision of the skin at the outer canthus for the eradication of "crow's feet." Am. J. Dermatol. Genitourin. Dis. 11:483, 1907.

37. Miller, C. C.: Subcutaneous section of the facial muscles to eradicate expression lines. Am. J. Surg. 21:235, 1907.

38. Miller, C. C.: Cosmetic surgery of the face. Int. J. Surg. 20:311, 1907.

39. Miller, C. C. and Miller, F.: Folds, bags and wrinkles of the skin about the eyes and their eradication by simple surgical methods. Med. Brief 35:540, 1907.

40. Miller, C. C.: Subcutaneous division of the fibers of the orbicularis muscle for overcoming "crow's feet". Med. Times (New York) 35:207, 1907.

41. Miller, C. C.: The Correction of Featural Imperfections, 2nd Ed. Oak Printing Company, Chicago, 1908.

42. Miller, C. C.: External canthotomy and section of the fibers of the orbicularis palpebrarum for minimizing "crow's feet". St. Louis Clin. 20:213 1907.

43. Miller, C. C.:The eradication by surgical means of the nasolabial line. Ther. Gaz. (Detroit) 23:676, (1907).

44. Miller, C. C.: The Care of Rupture by Paraffin Injections. Oak Printing Co., Chicago, 1908.

45. Miller, C. C.: The limitations and use of paraffin in cosmetic surgery. Wis. Med. Recorder 11:277, 1908.

46. Miller, C. C.: Cosmetic Surgery: The Correction of Featural Imperfections. F. A. Davis, Philadelphia, 1925.

47. Natvig, P.: Some aspects of the character and personality of Jacques Joseph. Plast. Reconstr. Surg. 47:452, 1971.

48. Noël, A.: La Chirurgie Esthétique: Son Rôle Social. Masson et Cie, Paris, 1926.

49. Noël, A.: Die ästhetische Chirurgie und ihre soziale Bedeutung. Johann Ambrosius Barth, Leipzig, 1932.

50. Passot, R.: La chirurgie esthétique des rides du visages. Presse Méd. 27:258, 1919.

51. Passot, R.: II. La correction chirurgicale des rides du visage. Bull. Acad. Méd. 82:112, 1919.

52. Regnault, P. and Stephenson, K. L.: Dr. Suzanne Noël: the first woman to do esthetic surgery. Plast. Reconstr. Surg. 48:133, 1971.

53. Robin, G.: Dr. Suzanne Noël. In Dictionnaire National des Contemporains, Vol. 1. La Jeunesse, Paris, 1936, p. 461.

54. Roe, J. O.: The deformity termed "pug nose" and its correction by a simple operation. Med. Rec. 31:621, 1887, reprinted in Plast. Reconstr. Surg. 45:78, 1970.

55. Roe, J. O.: The correction of angular deformities of the nose by a subcutaneous operation. Med. Rec. 40:57, 1891.

56. Rogers, B. O.: New Faces for Old After 40 Vol. 2., No. 2. Ciba Pharmaceutical Co., 1967.

57. Rogers, B. O.: Ely's 1881 operation for correction of protruding ears: a medical "first." Plast. Reconstr. Surg. 42:584, 1968.

58. Rogers, B. O.: Carl Ferdinand von Graefe (1787–1840). Plast. Reconstr. Surg. 46:554, 1970.

59. Rogers, B. O.: A chronologic history of cosmetic surgery. Bull. N. Y. Acad. Med. 47:265, 1971.

60. Rogers, B. O.: A brief history of cosmetic surgery. Surg. Clin. North Am. 51:265, 1971.

61. Rogers, B. O.: Early historical rhinoplasty. (In press.)

62. Shakespeare, W.: The Second part of Henrie the fourth, continuing to his death. . . . Printed by V. S. for Andrew Wise and William Aspley, London, 1600.

63. Szymanowski, von J.: Handbuch der operativen Chirurgie. Verlag Friedrich Vieweg und Sohn, Braunschweig, 1870.

Aesthetic Plastic Surgery 1:177-194, 1977
©1977 by Springer-Verlag New York Inc.

The History of Blepharoplasty to Correct Blepharochalasis

Kathryn L. Stephenson M.D.

Santa Barbara, California

Surgical relief of the full overhanging eyelid and of puffiness and wrinkling of the lower eye-lid was undertaken by Arabic surgeons of the tenth and eleventh centuries A.D. (Fig. 1) according to Sichel (59) writing in the Annales d'Oculistique. Sichel in 1844 was not the first French surgeon to have described these conditions, but with unusual scholarly integrity he referred to the earlier publications of Dupuytren (23).

Sichel's specific reference to Albucasis' work (1) is of historical interest. Abul Qasim (936–1013), or Albucasis as he is more commonly known, was born in the Andalusian town of Zahra near Cordova and was the author of a great medical-surgical treatise called the Al-Tas'rif (Fig. 2). The surgical part of the treatise survives in Channing's Arabic text and translation (Oxford, Clarendon Press, 1778) and was translated again in 1861 by Dr. Lucien Leclerc (1). In Volume II, Chapter 15, entitled "Cauterization for the Relaxation of the Eyelids," Albucasis wrote as follows:

> In the relaxation of the eyelids following illness or caused by fluid, it is necessary to cauterize one time with the semilunar cautery this form. If one wishes one can cauterize a little above the eyelids, two times on each side avoiding approaching the temples. The length of the cauterization will be the length of the eyelids. It is necessary to support with the hand the cautery and only burn one-third of the thickness of the skin.

Reference to this type of problem by Ali ibn-Isa (Jesu Haly) of Baghdad (3) (circa 940–1010 A.D.) in his memorandum book translated by Casey A. Wood is fascinating reading for the plastic surgeon as well as the ophthalmologist. Ophthalmology and optics were particularly advanced by the Arabic surgeons, of which Ali ibn-Isa was perhaps the most outstanding.

Ali ibn-Isa wrote of blepharoptosis, extraction of cataracts, corneal tattooing to facilitate the sale of slaves, excision of epidermoid cysts, and lagophthalmus. In the 31st chapter entitled "Relaxation (Ptosis) of the Upper Lid (Istirha)," he wrote the following:

> Blepharoptosis of the upper lid results from a relaxation (paralysis) so that it can no longer be raised. Often this enfeeblement is so marked that the lashes turn in and

Address reprint requests to Kathryn L. Stephenson, M.D., Surgical Medical Group Inc., 2235 Castillo Street, Santa Barbara, California 93105

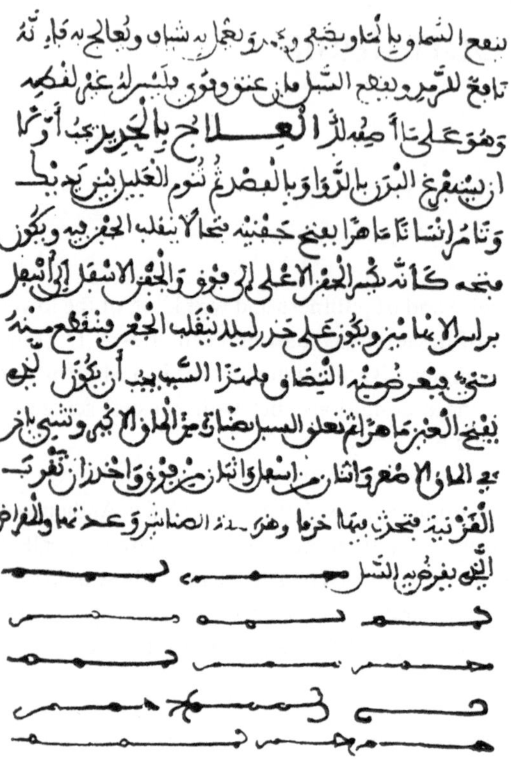

Fig. 1. Cauterization for relaxation of the eyelids and appropriate instruments. (From ref. 44.)

scratch the eyeball. The condition is due to excessive secretion of humors that in the lid gain the upper hand over normal complexion of the parts, just as the absence of a moist humor and a redundancy of dryness bring a hardening of the lid. In the treatment of ptosis the diet must be reduced and the patient forbidden moist food, such as milk and vegetables. The lid should be rubbed with desiccating and astringent agents like celadine, saffron, acacia, myrrh and myrtle water. If these simple remedies fail, resort to the measures I have described in Chapter X, on surgical elevation of the upper lid sometimes required in trichiasis.

His reference to the surgery described in Chapter X under trichiasis and its treatment is as follows:

Having put the patient to sleep, the lid must be everted so that the eyelashes can be firmly grasped between thumb and fingers on the left hand, which at the same time holds a spatula that presses out the middle of the eyelid. Then the lid margin must be split along its whole length with a small knife (qamadin). This should be carefully done, so that the whole incision lies evenly throughout the exact middle of the palpebral margin. If the incision is not made properly and there are irregularities at the

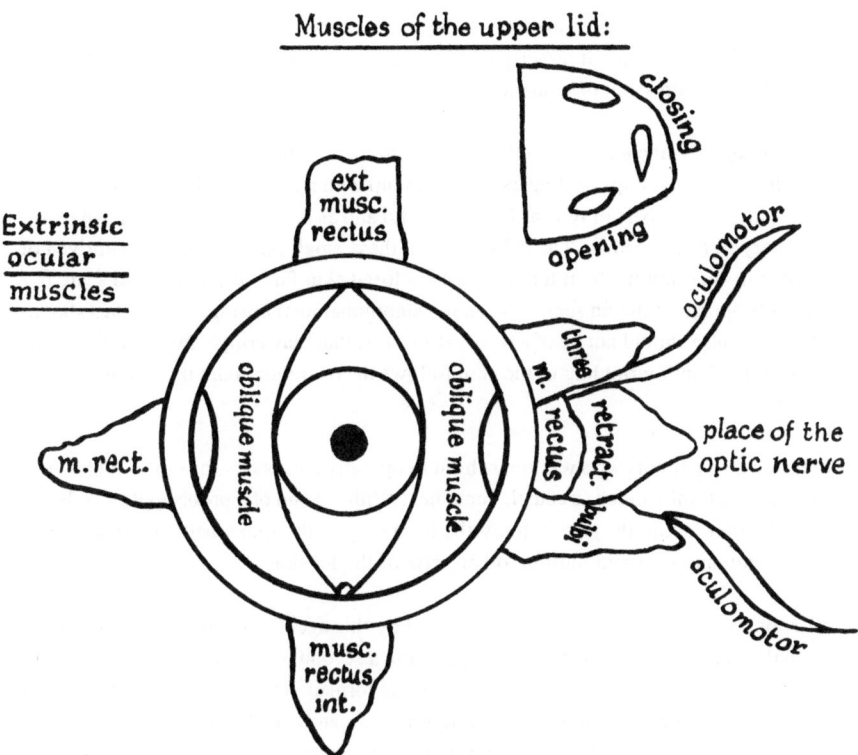

Fig. 2. The ocular muscles as shown by Hunain. (From Meyerhof's translation of the Ten Treatises, ref. 3.)

ends the central split will fail of its purpose. The next step is to carry out the folding (plication) of the lid tissue to be excised. Having determined the position and amount of these, conditioned largely upon the situation and number of false lashes, the latter are to be excised, cutting out most tissue where exuberant hairs are most numerous. To accomplish this, first enter three armed needles of a sharp trident through the lid at equidistant points and in a straight line. With these held in the left hand, elevate the lid and make the required excision with the right hand.

Note that the foregoing operation calls for experience, good judgment and operative skill.

The procedure should be carried out on the upper lid only, and the excision of the parts that lie beneath the introduced threads must be done with scissors.

Moreover it is wise to avoid a lagophthalmia, that the awakened patient should be asked to open and close both eyes before the chief or final excisions are made. The lips of the wound are now brought together with three equidistant stitches, the middle one to be tied first. The parts are now covered with yellow powder and a small bandage applied.

Many eye surgeons use a continuous suture, entering the needle in the lower margin of the wound so as to unite it directly with the edge that is next to the eyebrow. Some surgeons add a dressing of white lead ointment to the above mentioned powder.

More frequently one employs in these cases another method (tabin). Gather a fold of lid skin between a couple of fingers, or raise it up with a hook, and lay the fold between two small wooden bars or rods as long as the lid and as broad as the lancet. Bind their ends very tightly together. The skin between these small pieces of wood, deprived of nutriment, dies and in about ten days the enclosed skin falls off, leaving no scar. If after this operation the lid seems too short (lagophthalmus) astringent remedies should be used. These should not be of a desiccating sort, that may cripple the lid muscles. If, on the other hand, wrinkling of the skin follows the operation, both these remedies are in order.

In the case of patients who will not submit to operative measures, one must do his best by using such substitutes as caustic remedies. With the end of a probe apply a little of the cauterant (about the size of a myrthe leaf) only to the spot where you desire a contraction and so avoid burning other parts of the lid skin.

As soon as a local inflammation is produced by this agent, wipe off the medicament from the burned area and repeat the application a second or even a third time, until the skin of the part is burned black and a crust has formed. Then remove the caustic and dress the parts with a poultice or a mixture of wax and oil until the eschar drops. Finally, apply white lead ointment until cicatrization is complete.

Fragments of blepharoplastic techniques from the Middle Ages

Until the publication of Dupuytren (23) in 1839, there is a hiatus in ophthalmologic medical history because only fragments of the writings of ophthalmologists of that period are preserved. Dr. P. Pansier (54) collected and published these in 1903 in a volume entitled *Collectio Ophthalmologica Veterum Auctorum,* and in Fasc. I the works of Arnaldi de Villanova (1235–1311) and Johannis de Casso are presented. On page 262 of this text, under the title *De Relaxatione Palpebre et Cure Ejus,* the condition of hanging of the eyelids with inversion of the lashes that traumatize the eye is described, and, as in the Arabic texts, diets and desiccating applications were recommended. With the failure of these methods, it was recommended that finally one should resort to the method used in treatment of scrofula, and directions were given for opening the eyelid, retracting it with hooks, then excoriating the base, and finally closing the wound.

Nineteenth century plastic surgical techniques

Dupuytren's *Lecons Orales de Clinique Chirurgicale, Volume 3* page 376, as recorded by his students Brierre de Boismont and Marx in 1839, in translation reads as follows:

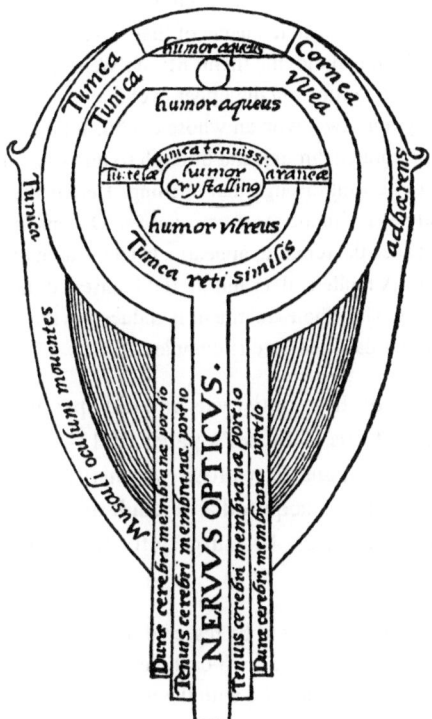

Fig. 3. The anatomy of the eye. (From ref. 3; Thesaurus of Alhazen Bale, 1572 A.D.)

Before leaving what is relative to the diseases of the ocular apparatus, we should say a few words about edema of the eyelids that, after having resisted all known means, produces such a slakening of the skin of that region in the long run, that it falls down in front of the eyeball and, more or less completely, interferes with vision. One encounters this curious disease among young girls of lymphatic constitution having white skin, blonde hair, and fleshy figures. As has been said, all internal therapeutic means and topical remedies praised in similar cases are ineffectual.

When he was consulted, on several occasions, for lesions of this type, Mr. Dupuytren thought that excision of a part of the distended skin would be succeeded by a cicatrice that would put an end to deformity.

The operation which one uses in this case is wholly analogous to the one used to remedy trichiasis. One does the same thing on the skin that is done on the conjunctiva when combatting certain invertings of the eyelid, and success is no less assured. It nevertheless happens that one first operation is insufficient, and we must return to it a second time. The cicatrice which forms soon ceases to be apparent. It conceals itself in the midst of the folds which form concentric curves on that movable part.

The eyelids can still be the seat of small encysted tumors that often develop in their thickness, and which the ancient authors designate with the name of 'hail stones'. Most surgeons counsel dissecting them and completely removing them. Mr. de Wenzel (one does not know why) says to make an incision vertical on the upper eyelid and horizontal on the lower eyelid. Mr. Dupuytren saw a woman whose eyelid, following the removal of a tumor of this kind, was perforated through and through so that when it was completely lowered the patient saw quite well through that opening. Here is the method he put into use for fifteen years, always with the same fine success: One inserts the left index finger beneath the eyelid to cause the tumor to appear; a lancet is used to open the area, one sees by this expression. A molten silver nitrate rod is inserted into the cyst, and is run over its internal surface. The whole treatment is reduced to that; wash with fresh water and at the end of eight days the cure is complete.

Thus we learn that the older surgeons were aware of these fatty cysts and did operate to remove them as did Sichel. Particularly significant to us is Sichel's paper of 1844 (59) distinguishing betweeen paralytic ptosis, atonique ptosis, and fatty ptosis. Atonique ptosis he described as a malady sometimes congenital, sometimes acquired as a result of chronic edema or prolonged use of creams and/or of unknown causes. His surgery for this condition he described as follows:

When one has well calculated the extent of the fragment to be resected, one can introduce at its face under this small clamp which is fixed, two or three small silk sutures placed parallel and vertically. One can take this fold with the use of curved scissors and tie the threads to establish a suture.

He then described a third type of ptosis which he stated to be a modification of the preceding one, referred to as fatty ptosis.

It is produced by a certain quantity of fat deposited between the skin and the orbicularis muscle. This fat is most often in continuity with the cellular orbital adipose tissue which separates the fibers of the orbicularis muscle and penetrates between them under the skin. Most often this fat is situated under the muscle and after the ablation of a fold of fat it is necessary to incise transversely and parallel in the direction of these fibers to demonstrate the tumor and elevate it. The characteristics of this affliction are the same as those of atonic ptosis except that instead of being laxed, flaccid and wrinkled, the eyeball is on the contrary flaccid and swollen and presents a tumor sometimes even a bit elastic under the finger. Most ordinarily this tumor is encircled between the border adhering to the eyeball and its wide transversal fold. Often it hangs in front of the inferior part of the eyelid in the form of a bulge or of weighty transversal sac which more than a simple fold of skin renders movements of the eyelid more difficult.

Sichel agreed with the Arabs that it is a malady which cannot be cured without operation. He had operated for this condition several times.

Merkel (43), in an 1874 report included in the *Graefe und Saemisch Handbuch der Ges. Augenheilkunde,* regarded the bulging out of the area of skin between the tarsal plate and orbital rim as the result of atrophy of the orbital septum. He has shown it was in no way dissimilar to atrophy of all the other fascia in the older individual. Therefore, the septum was unable to hold back the orbital fat as formerly. Alibert in 1832 (2) Graf in 1836 (30), Von Ammon and Baumgarten in 1842 (4), and others noting the condition of the overhanging eyelid suggested only excision of the skin. Arlt (1877) (6), however, described the condition as ptosis adiposia which was seen in young people and occasionally in older people, in which the upper eyelid appeared to be enlarged and hung down although it did not press against the globe. He noted that when picking up a fold of this thin and pliant skin, one found soft elastic skin underneath, much like the fatty tissue of the orbit. This was pushed out so much that one had to take away a good portion of it with the scissors in order to suture the wound satisfactorily. He also noted that the skin to be excised did not need to be over 10 mm in width, but to obtain a satisfactory cosmetic result it was necessary to extend the incision from the outer orbit to above the tear duct.

Hotz in 1880 (34) was aware not only of the writings of MacKenzie (1854) (42), Arlt (6) and Von Ammon and Baumgarten (4), who called the condition

"epiblepharon," but also, of Sichel's work (59) and the condition he described as ptosis atonique. Hotz, however, attributed this problem to prolapse of the skin, stating:

> In order to obtain the proper result, I had to think both of the functional and the cosmetic effect of the surgery. This was very difficult for me to achieve if the skin of the upper rim is tarsus. I felt that if you connected the skin with the upper rim of the tarsus then the skin of the upper and lower portion of the eyelid is stabilized then all of the movements could follow the natural course, so that the skin of the upper lid could grow together like the surgery I described for entropion and I would like to try this technique because in my opinion this condition is a prolapse of the lid skin and muscles.

His operation he described as follows:

> On September 16th, under Chloroform anesthesia, I performed the following surgery, I made an incision from a point 2 mm. above the tear duct, extending the convexity of the upper lid rim. I excised a wide enough strip so that I could free the tendon of the palpebral levator muscle, the middle third of the wound I took two deep sutures. With these two deep sutures I attached the skin of the lid to the skin rim so I could connect the skin directly with the tarsus because on both the medial and lateral portions of the tarsus the skin was especially lax.

Fuchs (1896) (27) also referred to Von Ammon's and Sichel's works stating that his own case was similar to that referred to by Von Ammon and Baumgarten as epiblepharon and Sichel as ptosis atonicque. He became involved in describing and naming the condition "blepharochalasis." For this condition, he preferred the surgery of Hotz but stated that the success of the operation decreased with the passage of time. Fuchs actually contributed nothing toward an understanding of the problem, but apparently he had such prestige that he is often quoted.

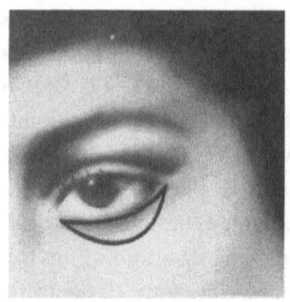

Fig. 4. Line of incision in the operation below the eye. Crescent of skin is entirely removed. Size of the crescent varies according to the amount of bagging, folding, or wrinkling of the skin. Above the eye the area of skin removed varies in shape, the operator simply picking up and cutting away the excess. (From ref. 46.)

Clinically, Schmidt-Rimpler (58) noted that after edematous infiltration of the eyelid regressed either spontaneously or after packing, the skin of the upper eyelids was covered with numerous small wrinkles. He concluded that the bulge was due to abnormal fat collection and therefore surgery was undertaken, and he noted that under the bulge there was a defect in the musculature through which the orbital fat covered with fascia appeared. Therefore, he incised the fascia and the fat rolled out. Through slight pressure one could empty almost any amount at will. He resected the fat and the musculature and then sutured muscle and skin. Following this he had an excess wrinkling of the skin. He noted that this condition was fairly normal for older people and gave credit to Merkel for having noted that the bulging of the are of skin between the tarsal plate and the orbital rim resulted from atrophy of all the fascia, therefore the orbital septum had lost its strength and was no longer able to retain the orbital fat in its normal position. He concluded that his case, which occurred in a younger person, was due to congenital weakness of the fascia, and he felt that "fat hernia" was a term that could be justifiably used to describe the condition.

In 1906 Bach (8) observed the fluctuant character of the upper eyelid, and after removing a piece of skin as in blepharochalasis he noted that the tense and slightly separated muscle bundles of the orbicularis were evident; underneath there was a fascia-like membrane which he incised at the temporal side with the result that fat protruded immediately. He removed this fat and proceeded to open the medial end of the membrane where he found nothing but empty space and concluded, "In the future one would have to incise the membrane under the muscle to determine the fact whether there is a fat collection in the upper lids with 'blepharochalasis'. To determine whether the possible fat collection represents a hernia of the orbital fat or not the behavior or position of the tarsal orbital fascia would have to always be examined."

Sporadically, ophthalmologists Weidler (63), Rohmer (56), and others noted the importance of this bulging fat and recommended removal of the fat for the correction of this condition. As previously, most of the ophthalmologists and surgeons were concerned with the etiology of this disease and often thought the skin changes to be primary rather than secondary as a result of bulging of the fat. They also were concerned with trying to differentiate this type of eyelid pouching from some systematic disease or endocrine change.

Improvements in blepharoplasty by twentieth century plastic surgeons

With renewed interest in cosmetic rather than functional problems, blepharoplasty became the interest of the plastic surgeons Miller (1907) (46), Kolle (1911) (38), Noel (1926) (50) (Fig. 5), and Hunt (1926) (35) (Fig. 6).

In surgery of the upper eyelid, Miller considered it preferable to have the line of incision follow the convexity of the tarsal margin, but he also thought that certain cases could be operated to better advantage by removing the skin from the upper lid forming a line of union close to the free margin of the lid. He further thought it necessary to extend the excision in the outer canthal area. His admonitions with regard to undertaking this type surgery are of interest. In his intial paper (46) he wrote:

> These conditions may be easily overcome by simpl surgical procedures, which are performed painlessly. By painlessly, I do not mean that the patient is hanging on to the table with both hands and praying for the early conclusion of the ordeal.

In 1925 Miller (49) wrote:

> It is well worthwhile to consider the blood of the patient. While the amount lost may not be important from the standpoint of the health of the patient, even if particular efforts were not made to prevent such loss, the effect on the patient of such

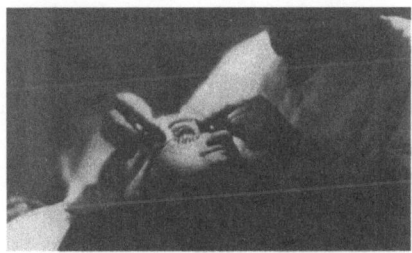
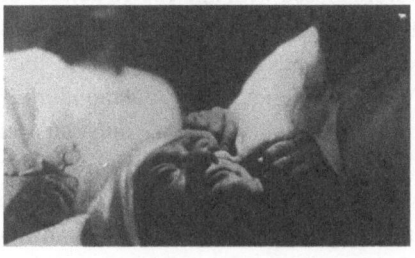

Fig. 5. Madame A. Noel performing a blepharoplasty. (From ref. 50.)

31

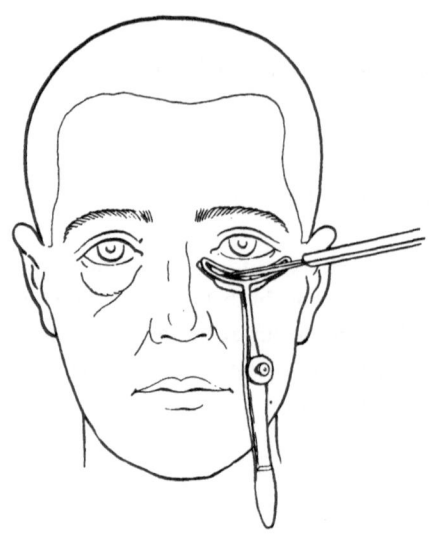

Fig. 6. Hunt's method of removing redundant skin (lid rhytidectomy of the eyelid by use of author's clamp). These are similar to fine silver clips used by A. Noel and illustrated in her publication of 1926. (From ref. 35.)

conservation is very good. It robs them of much of the nervousness that naturally is felt while undergoing operation. Nine-tenths of the women who submit to these operations are highstrung, modern types who suffer from enough nerves. Operation is dreaded by them but they are so anxious to secure the effects of operations that they submit even though the surgery is likely to be a severe test for them.

To avoid these ill effects too much surgical display should be avoided by the surgeon. The room where the operation is to be performed need not be elaborately equipped. A few simple instruments only are used in operation. These may be placed between two towels on a small table. One assistant only is needed by the surgeon. Several people bustling about getting in each other's way is only a nuisance anyhow. When the operation is painless and bloodless and the patient is alone with two calm, unhurried people there is nothing to terrify and add a psychic trauma to tense nerves.

Dr. Miller performed his surgery under 2 to 4% novocaine in order to avoid bulging the tissues excessively. He controlled bleeding by pressure and the application of hemostats. He used a knife for his initial incision. The wounds were closed with interrupted sutures of fine slik or cambric, and the sutures were tied lightly. He removed the sutures within 2 to 3 days and supported the wound by collodion gauze strips placed beneath the suture line. The avoid eversion of the lower lid, he illustrated V-shaped angles at each outer and inner canthal area. To correct eversion, Miller advised multiple small wedges as illustrated in Figure 7.

In 1928 Bourguet (15) wrote his influential treatise *Poches Sous Les Yeux,* in which he described the anatomy of the orbital cavity in detail emphasizing the fibrous expansion around the muscle which maintains the fat within the cavity. When there was an increase in the weight and volume of the fat, however, it was permitted to penetrate between the muscles and out beneath the attenuated orbicularis, forming fatty packets. Bourguet stated:

> The orbital cavity is filled with a vast adipose layer, a layer of padding within which pass the muscles of the eyeball. It can be divided into two parts; one is contained in the muscular funnel that goes from the bottom of the orbit to the posterior hemisphere of the eye: the other is situated above and contained, consequently, between the muscles and the orbital wall. It is this latter which will interest us. This adipose mass is enclosed like the "Boule de Bichat" in a thin conjunctive capsule attached to the periosteum by membraneous, easily torn prolongations. It comes to abut against the orbital septum and pushes it forward in many cases, giving rise to a sort of bloating underneath the tarsal cartilage in the form of a cross, quite marked, especially on the lower eyelid. It is not, as is generally thought, due to edema, but to a fatty hernia. How is it produced and at what points can it appear?
>
> Let us suppose that the two eyelids are lifted and the fat drawn delicately back, so as to have before us the base of the orbital cavity and its contents. Precisely in the middle we notice the ocular globe, on which the straight muscles arrive to insert themselves at its four principal points.
>
> The sheath of the right internal gives off a fibrous, rectangular expansion that goes to be inserted within, on the crest of the Unguis; it is the internal alaron. The sheath of the right external supplies a similar expansion, the inserted part of which is affixed externally by an enlarged base to the orbital wall and to the external palpebral ligament; it is the external alaron. These two alarons are strengthened by other fibers, above and below, which come—for the upper half—from the external and internal borders of the right superior muscle, levator of the eyelid, and—for the lower half—from the internal and external borders of the lower small oblique muscle. They form, then, concentric fibers all around the ocular globe, all of which together has been designated under the name of suspensor ligament of the eye, by certain anatomists.
>
> It is still to be noted that other fibers become detached from the external border of the small oblique muscle to go to implant themselves on the lower external corner of the edge of the orbit, becoming part of the large ligament.
>
> Thus if we examine fig. 1 [Fig. 8] we realize that there are some emptinesses in certain places. Fatty hernias pass through there. We see two of them above; one is found placed between the internal alaron and the pulley of the large oblique, and the other is between that pulley and the internal border of the lacrymal gland. Three of them are below; the first is contained between the internal alaron and the small oblique, the second between this muscle and its bow-shaped expansions, and the third is bound by these same fibers and the external alaron.

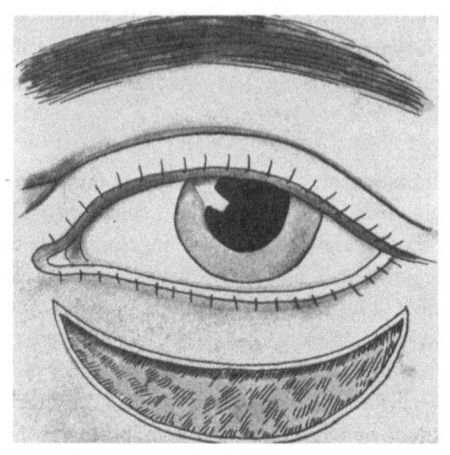
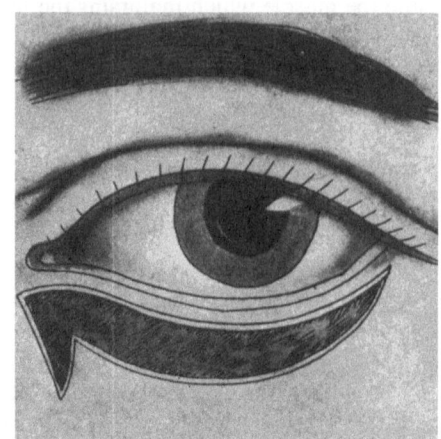
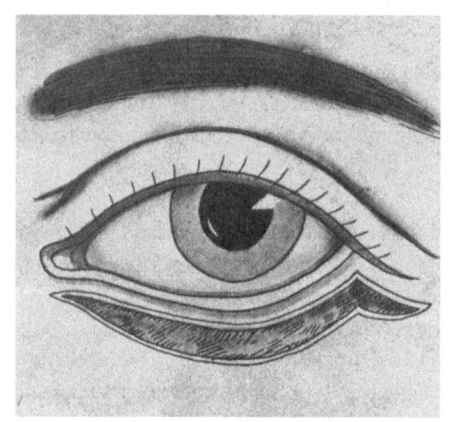
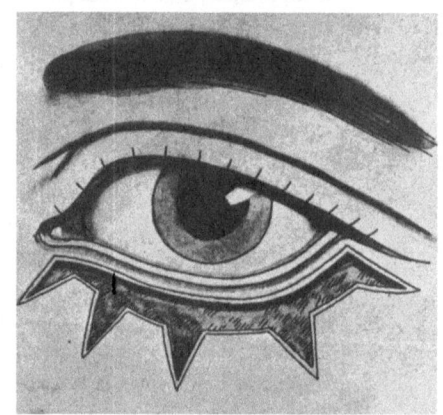
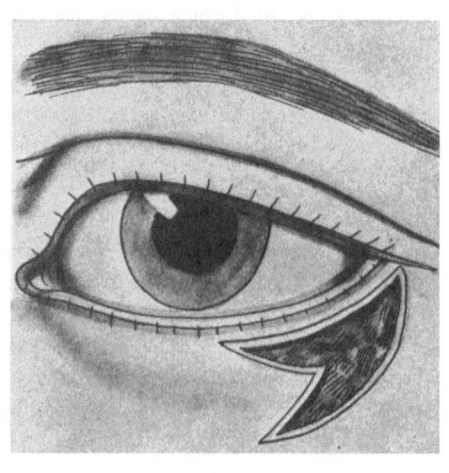
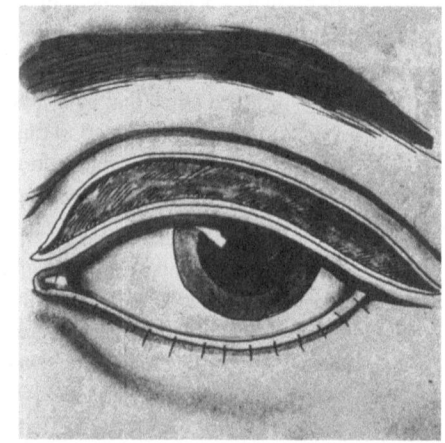

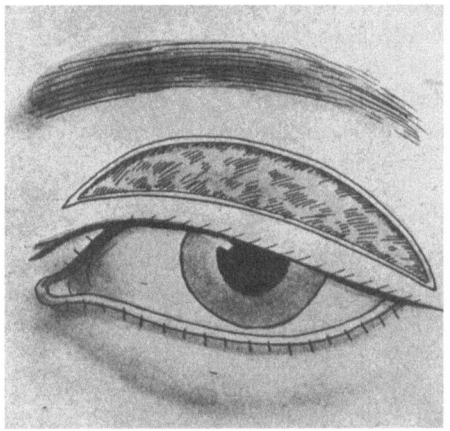 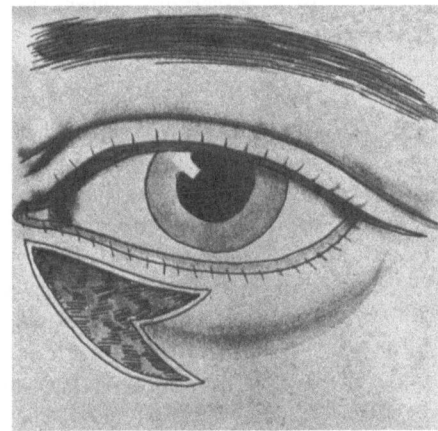

Fig. 7. Illustrations of types of excision of lid tissue recommended by C. C. Miller for various conditions. (From ref. 49.)

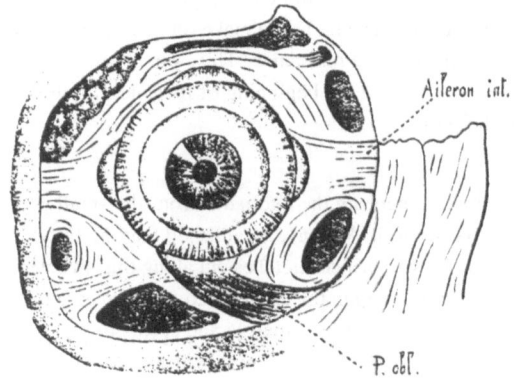

Fig. 8. Bourguet's illustration of areas through which fatty tissue hernias extrude. (From ref. 15.)

We believe that these adipose orifices, through which certain vessels and nerves escape as well are very narrow or do not exist to speak of in the subjects who do not exhibit these palpebral baginesses, for among them the suspensor ligament of the eye is very developed, whereas among others, on the contrary, all the fibers are less expanded and these spaces are quite large. These "pouches" are not the infirmities of old age. We have noticed them among relatively young persons and they stand out, of course, with age.

We have noticed, however, an isolated hernial point for each orifice. We have found, for example, a nernia, single or associated above the lacrimal sac passing through the orifice located between the internal alaron and the reflexion pulley of the large oblique.

35

We have seen also another evagination beneath the internal alaron and another above the levator muscle of the upper eyelid. Finally, in a certain number of cases one may see, admirably, that the lower eyelid, pushed back below the tarsal cartilage, is so slightly constricted on the outside. This constricture is due to the bow-shaped fibers of the small oblique muscle, which seems to place a kind of rein on this adipose protrusion, marking the eyelid with a groove going from top to bottom and from the inside to the outside.

Lastly, when the fatty bulge is very pronounced, this groove is lacking. There is then a veritable "garland" stretching (with regard to the lower eyelid) from one commissure to another. These palpebral projections, at least at the onset of their appearance, thrust beneath the skin in a manner that varies with the days or even with certain hours of the day. We have noted this phenomenon in particular in respect to the hernia which is found located between the pulley of the large oblique and the internal alaron. It goes in or out in the morning, is scarcely visible during the day, and projects, or vice versa, in the evening, as a fairly large cyst does and having the shape of a kidney bean.

In the orbital cavity there are many arterial and venous vessels. When, on account of an action of the vasomotors, the vessels distend to let more blood pass, an increase in the volume of the content of that cavity results. The fat has to make room since there is filling tissue, and to escape through points of least resistance. This, we assert, is the reason for which we do or do not see—at least at the beginning of its genesis—this hernia of the upper internal part of the orbit.

With regard to the thrust that occurs below, beneath the internal alaron, the small oblique muscle does not constitute a barrier to it. We have established that the fatty pouch which escapes through the internal lower orifice stretches out along this muscle, covers it, overflows, and comes to attach itself upon the fatty pouch adjacent, which goes out through the other orifice located outside of this muscle and seems to become an intergal part of this second pouch. These two extensions of fat clasp the small oblique muscle like a cloth hung on a cord.

With a less scholarly approach than that of Sichel, Bourguet stated that he had found no previous publication concerning the operation for the removal of fat.

Our operation. We first published our operating technique at the Academie de Medecine de Paris in November, 1925. We presented patients to the Societe de Medecine de Paris in February, 1926. We have not found any publication previous to ours concerning this method of treatment. As with every hernia operation, one must come upon the [protruding] herniated organ, open the sac in which it is contained, force it back into the cavity if it is a part of the intestinal tract, from which it has come out, or resect it if there is an epiploic fringe, and lastly remove the sac. This is nearly the same procedure which we followed to treat surgically the "pouches under the eyes".

After local anesthesia we make an incision in the bottom of the lower conjunctival sac, and after cutting the muscle of Muller we come to the hernia, onto the hernial sac which we free over its whole area. This done, the protrusion is even more considerable. We transfix it from top to bottom with U-shaped stitches and with catgut collargole 000.

This phase executed, we excise all the part of the sac whose contents extends beyond the orbital edge. The catguts are then knotted and the sac closed. In front we restore a wall with the fibers which are around the orifices. It has happened to us many times when we realized that the ti sue of the orbital septum was too loose, that as a second procedure made a cutaneous external incision as a procedure beneath the tarsal cartilage, to reinforce it, doing as the Mayo brothers for umbilical hernias.

When protrusions which are located on the upper lid are concerned, the incisions are cutaneous for it is impossible for us to go through the bottom of the upper conjunctival sac, which is too deep. We have to go across the large ligament and we do then as we would for hernias seated on the lower eyelids.

He then illustrated his results by pre- and postoperative photographs.

The work of Bourguet was popularized rapidly. Passot (55) and several others continued to follow Bourguet's recommendation of the transconjunctival apporach to the lower lid. However, the technique advocated and explicitly described by Madame Noel became the more standardized approach. In her paper of 1928 (51) (Fig. 9), she described her technique for correcting the flaccid eyelid, the eylid with fat, and the eyelid with wrinkled skin only. She limited the quantity of skin to be resected by the use of a small silver serrated clamp with three teeth, which she applied prior to injecting the anesthesia, and then excised the tissue by use of the scissors. She recommended excision of the skin 2 mm below the lashes for the lower eyelid. She recognized that further injection of anesthesia might be necessitated when fat was removed from the sac fragment by fragment.

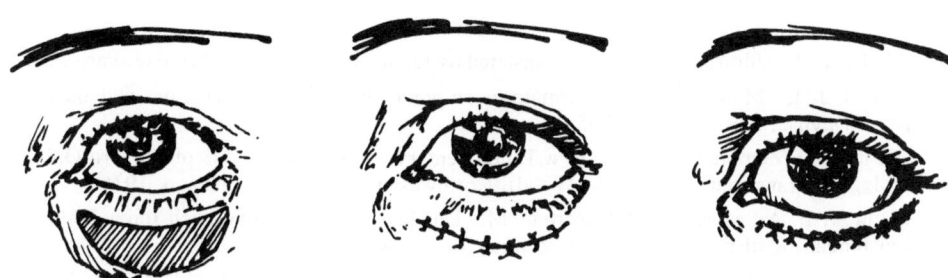

Fig. 9. Blepharoplasty incision illustrated in a monograph by Madame Noel (from ref. 51).

There have been some variations in the technique in subsequent years, but the design of the external excision as illustrated in Joseph's (36) text of 1931 was established (Fig. 10).

By 1930 an idealized form of the eye and eyelid region for Caucasians could be obtained or maintained by the previously described techniques, and could be accentuated by the elaborate use of cosmetics. The "baggy eye" previously associated with so-called indiscretions both from the use of alcohol and from questionable sexual excesses no longer had to be endured.

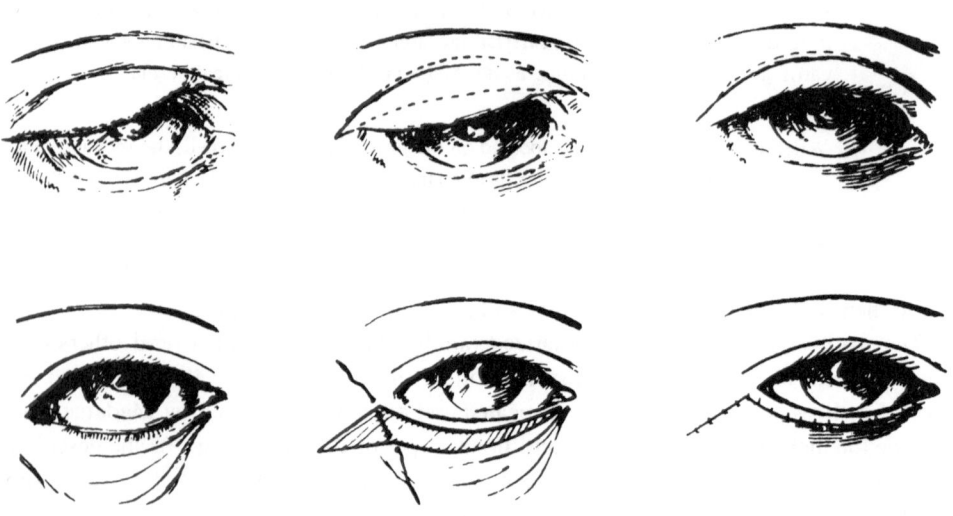

Fig. 10. Outline of skin incisions for removal of excess eyelid tissue (from ref. 36).

References

1. Abulcasis: La chirurgie d'abulcasis (translated by Lucien Leclerc). J. B. Baillière, Paris, 1861.
2. Alibert, J. L.: Monographie des dermatoses ou précis théorique et pratique des maladies de la peau. Daynac, Paris, 1832, p. 795.
3. Ali ibn-Isa: Memorandum Book of a Tenth-Century Oculist for the Use of Modern Ophthalmologists (translated by Casey A. Wood). Northwestern University, Chicago, 1936.
4. Ammon, F. A., von, and Baumgarten, M.: Die Plastische Chirurgie nach Ihren Bisherigen Leistungen, Kritisch Dargestellt. G. Reimer. Berlin. 842.
5. Angelucci, A.:Un cas de blepharochalazis. Ann. Ottamol. Clin. Occulista 34:842–843, 1905.
6. Arlt, C.: In: Graefe-Saemisch Handbuch Ges. Augenh., 1. Aufl. 2: 454, 1877.
7. Ascher, K. W.: Blepharochalasis mit Struma und Doppellippe. Klin. Monat. Augenheil. 65.86–96, 1920.

8. Bach, L.: Über symmetrische Lipomatosis der Oberlider (Blepharochalasis?). Arch. Augenh. 73:73–84, 1906.

9. Beck, J.: Plastic surgery about the face, head and neck. J. Indiana State Med. Assoc. 18:167, 1925.

10. Bedell, A. J.: Editorial comment. J.A.M.A. 61:1133, 1913.

11. Benedict, W. L.: Blepharochalasis: Report of three cases. J.A.M.A. 87:1735–1739, 1926.

12. Bettman, A. G.: Plastic surgery about the eyes. Ann. Surg. 88:994–1006, 1928.

13. Black, M.: A case of blepharochalasis. Ann. Ophthalmol. 24:404–407, 1915.

14. Bourguet, J.: La chirurgie esthétique de la face. Concours Médical pp. 1657–1670, 1921.

15. Bourguet, J.: Notre traitement chirurgical de "poches" sous les yeux sans cicatrice. Arch. Fr. Belg. Chir. 31:133, 1928.

16. Bulfill, A. P.: Blepharoptosis. Arch. Oftalmol. Hisp. Am. Barcelona 7:696–701, 1907.

17. Chiarini, P.: Sopra un caso di blepharo-calasi. Boll. d'Ocul. Firenza 18, 1896.

18. Dalen, A.: Ein Fall von Blepharochalasis. Mitteilungen aus des Augenklinik des Carolinischen Chirurgischen, Stockholm, Heft IV, 1902.

19. De Berardinis, D.: Blefaracalasis. Ann Di'Ottal Pavia 34:841–843, 1905.

20. Denonvilliers, C.P.: Blepharoplastie. Bull. Soc. Chir. 7:243, 1856.

21. Desselaers: Rev. Espan. Med. Cir. 119, 1928.

22. Dunn, J.: Symmetrical falling of the skin of the upper yelids. Richmond J. Practice 10:75–77, 1896.

23. Dupuytren, M.: Leçons orales de clinique chirurgicale, 2nd Ed., Vol. 3. Germer-Baillière, Paris, 1839, pp. 377–378.

24. Eitner, E.: Indications and technic of cosmetic correction of facial wrinkles. Wien. Klin. Wochenschr. 41:1281, 1928.

25. Elschnig, A.: Fetthernien, sog. "Tränensäcke" der Unterlider. Klin. Monatsbl. Augenh. 84:763–766, 1930.

26. Fruhwald, V.: Über einen Fall von Hängewange behoben durch eine Modifikation der Josephschen Operation. Wien. Klin. Wochenschr. 72:1336–1337, 1922.

27. Fuchs, E.: Über Blepharochalasis (Erschlaffung der Lidhaut). Wien. Klin. Wochenschr. 9:109, 1896.

28. Fuchs, E.: Textbook of Ophthalmology, 8th Ed. (translated by A. Duane). J. B. Lippincott Co., Philadelphia, 1924.

29. Fuchs, E.: Diseases of the Eye, 10th Ed. (translated by E. V. L. Brown). J. B. Lippincott Co., Philadelphia, 1932.

30. Graf, D.: Örtliche erbliche Erschlaffung der Haut. Wochenschr. Ges. Heilkunde 2:97–100, 1836.

31. Heckel, E.: Blepharochalasis with ptosis: Report of a case. Am. J. Ophthalmol. 4:273–275, 1921.

32. Hirsch, A.: Bibliographisches Lexicon der hervorrag. Aerzte 1:235, 1880.

33. Hirschberg, J.: Arabian ophthalmology. J.A.M.A. 45:1127–1131, 1905.

34. Hotz, F.: Über das Wesen und die Operation der sogenannten Ptosis Atonica. Arch. Augenheilk 9:95–101, 1880.

35. Hunt, H. L.: Plastic Surgery of the Head, Face and Neck. Lea & Febiger, Philadelphia, 1926.

36. Joseph, J.: Nasenplastik und sonstige Gesichtsplastik nebst Mammaplastik. Curt Kabitzsche, Leipzig, 1931.

37. Kestenbaum, A.: Wien. Med. Wochenschr. 37, 1928.

38. Kolle, F.: Plastic and Cosmetic Surgery. D. Appleton and Co., New York, 1911.

39. Kromeyer, F.: Die Behandlung der kosmetischen Hautleiden. Verlag G. Thieme, Leipzig, 1923.

40. Lexer, E.: Zur Gesichtsplastik. Arch. Clin. Chir. 92:749–793, 1910.

41. Lowenstein, A.: Andere Lidoperationen: Augenärztliche Operationslehre. In: Graefe und Saemisch Handbuch Ges. Augenheilkunde, 1922.

42. MacKenzie: Practical Treatise on the Diseases of the Eye, 4th Ed. Longman, London, 1854, p. 187.

43. Merkel, F.: In: Graefe und Saemisch Handbuch der ges. Augenheilkunde, Vol. I, 1874, p. 454.

44. Meyerhof, M.: Le guide d'oculistique . . . Mohammad ibn Qassoûm ibn Aslam Al-Ghâfiqî. Masnou, Barcelona, 1933.

45. Meyerhof, M.: Correspondence. N. Engl. J. Med. 233:79–80, 1945.

46. Miller, C. C.: Folds, bags and wrinkles of the skin about the eyes and their eradication by simple surgical methods. Med. Brief 35:540, 1907.

47. Miller, C. C.: Cosmetic Surgery, 2nd Ed. Oak Printing Co., Chicago, 1908.

48. Mller, C. C.: Subcutaneous section of the corrugator supercilii and of fibers of the orbicularis palpebarum. Long Island Med. J. 2:66, 1908.

49. Miller, C. C.: Cosmetic Surgery: the Correction of Featural Imperfections. F. A. Davis Co., Philadelphia, 1925.

50. Noel, A.: La chirurgie esthétique; son rôle social. Masson et Cie, Paris, 1926.

51. Noel, A.: La chirurgie esthétique. Imprimerie Thiron et Cie, Clermont (Oise), 1928.

52. Nutting, R. J.: Plastic surgery in and about the eyelids. Calif. State J. Med. 20:15–16, 1922.

53. Panas, P.: Thèse de Paris, 1873. Arch. Ophthalmol. 208, 1882.

54. Pansier, P.: Collectio Ophthalmologica Veterum Auctorum, Fasc. I. Arnaldi de Villanova, Editus circa annum 1308 and Johannis de Casso, Editus anno 1346. Librairie J. B. Baillière et Fils, Paris, 1903.

55. Passot, R.: La chirurgie esthétique pure: technique et résultats. G. Doin et Cie, Paris, 1931.

56. Rohmer, A.: Angio-mégalie symmétrique des paupières supérieures. Arch. Ophthalmol. 20: 407, 1900.

57. Schlaepfer, J.: Plastic operations on the face. Schweiz. Med. Wochenschr. 52:383–386, 1922.

58. Schmidt-Rimpler, J.: Fett-Hernien der oberen Augenlider. Centralbl. Prak. Augenh. 23:297–298, 1899.

59. Sichel, A.: Aphorismes pratiques sur divers points d'ophthalmologie. Ann. Ocul. 12:185–190, 1844.

60. Stein, R.: Indikation und Technik kosmetischer Faltenkorrekturen im Gesichte. Wien Clin. Wochenschr. 40:1168–1172, 1927.

61. Stein, R.: Blepharochalasis des Unterlides. Klin. Monatsbl. Augenh. 84:846–851, 1930.

62. Verhoff, F., and Friedenwald, J.: Blepharochalasis. Arch. Ophthalmol. 51:554–559, 1922.

63. Weidler, W.: Blepharochalasis: Report of 2 cases with the microscopic examination. J.A.M.A. 61:1128–1132, 1913.

The History of Rhytidectomy

Mario González-Ulloa M.D.

Mexico City, Mexico

Operations to counteract the process of aging have been directed mainly to the removal of facial wrinkles. Hence the term rhytidectomy (Greek *ritis,* wrinkle, and *ektomi,* excision). The present technical status of such operations is due to the combination of two forces. One is the constant, and constantly powerful, motive of vital men and women of every era to keep their facial and bodily appearance in youthful harmony with their inner feelings of strength and their vigor in action. The other is the progressive evolution of human thought and technical ability.

From a technical point of view, it is possible to discern a line of evolution from the first attempts at rhytidectomy published about the turn of the century down to the present status of total, sectional, and segmental rhytidectomy. Abstracting from numerous regressions and disregarding a multitude of variations, the major stages we shall chronicle are these: The first techniques published involved simple and local small excisions of skin about the hairline and in front of the ear; the skin was sutured without undermining. Somewhat later, the areas of excision grew slightly larger, and local undermining was essayed. A third major step was taken when the larger incisions coalesced into a single line stretching from above the patient's ear around the curve of the lobe, then upward and again backward at some distance from the occipital hairline. Once the safety and aesthetic success of the bolder incision were consolidated, attention was focused on more extensive undermining, reaching as far as the buccolabial sulcus and the mandibular line, and on more ingenious ways of camouflaging the scars. It was found that more permanent results were forthcoming if the excess adipose was removed and sutures on the aponeurosis were made when necessary, thus avoiding the tension of skin sutured purely to skin. The excision of a "Roman U"-shaped area of skin above and behind the ear was a precursor of the use of traction triangles in the mastoid and parietal regions for

0364-216X/80/0004-0001 $09.00

© 1980 Springer-Verlag New York Inc.

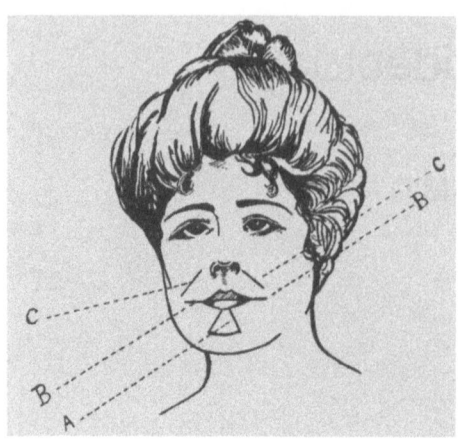

Fig. 1. Charles Conrad Miller eradicated wrinkles by subcutaneously sectioning the facial muscles. **A** Section of labial muscles below. **B** Lines of section of the orbicularis oris. **C** Lines of section of the fibers responsible for the buccolabial fold. Fig. 1 from [90], reproduced with permission

superior elevation and more enduring tension in the frontal and cervical areas. These various methods came to be not only advantageously combined, but also conveniently differentiated, so that at present the problems of the aging face can either be well treated integrally or with fine discrimination to broad regional or local segmental requirements.

The Precursors of Rhytidectomy

General interest in the etiology of wrinkling precedes by only a few years the first description, by Cantrell [23] and Cabanès [21], of some fragmentary techniques to eliminate wrinkles. Credit of priority, however, properly goes to Charles Conrad Miller [89, 90, 106] for his publication in 1907 of the details of serious surgical means for eradicating wrinkles (Fig. 1). He gave express attention to the buccolabial sulcus. His proposal was a subcutaneous sectioning of the facial muscles or, from inside the mouth, a more thorough correction though with greater risk of infection and reduced opportunity of precision. With a view to minimum visibility of the scar, Miller advised that the external incision should take place at the point where a dimple would form, if indeed one did not already exist.

Miller was no votary of the crude use of paraffin to replace adipose tissue absorbed in the aging process. No doubt to prevent all possibility of the danger that paraffin might have allowed eventual loss of shape, he relied on bits of braided silk, particles of celluloid, vegetable ivory, and gutta-percha.[1] In his recent article on the history of cosmetic surgery, Rogers [106] comments that Miller was "something of a quack and at the same time something of a surgical visionary."

The career of Eugen Holländer illustrates the evolution of antiaging techniques within the experience of a single man. Dissatisfied with the results of

---

[1] His successors have not followed him in this.

excising a plurality of small pieces of skin in front of the ear and in the border of the scalp, he gradually undertook a more ambitious procedure. He made a long vertical incision in front of the ear that then swung upward and laterally into the neck. From the temporal region of the face in front of the vertical line, removal of a crescent-shaped strip of skin, sometimes as much as 5 cm wide, allowed substantial elevation even without undermining [65, 106].

The Pioneer Period

Not all the pioneers of rhytidectomy spread their innovations through publication; some were teachers instead of writers. Sooner or later, however, those they taught began to write. Giving credit to his masters, Pozzi and Morestin, as well as to Mlle. Pertat, Raymond Passot [98] in 1919 described the following technique for eliminating cheek wrinkles and the buccolabial sulcus (Fig. 2): First, he began the operation by "withdrawing minuscule amounts of tegument in the preauricular region, using as a limit the lower part of the male's sideburns and the region onto which the mass of the female's long hair falls."[2] The calculation of the amount of skin to be resected was accomplished by performing the pinch maneuver, which was deployed in front of and above the tragus; the use of guidelines for the incision, drawn with a "dermographic pencil," marked out the ellipses characteristic of Passot's technique.

The skin segment resection was done under local anesthesia. Passot believed that a basic condition for producing ascent of the cheek tegument was the detachment of the adipose tissue down to the aponeurosis.

In order not to injure the facial branch of the orbicularis oculi, it is important to extract the cellulo-adipose [adipose tissue] cautiously in a separate operation from the one in which the dermis is resected.

The suture is done in separate stitches using horsehair.

If the resection is to be a large one, two or three consecutive sessions are suggested; a single operating period would result in a stretched suture line.

For correction of "crow's feet," small forceps in the temporal region, behind and over the external angle of the eye, are recommended. Ascending folds are thus eliminated. Opposite traction in front of the tragus eliminates the descending folds.

For the double chin, Passot recommended "an incision on the normal fold of the neck formed in the very limits of the suprahyoid and infrahyoid regions."

In the same year (1919), Julien Bourguet [10] differentiated among various areas and types of wrinkling; he promoted appropriately different techniques for the correction of each. For frontal wrinkling, he prescribed two crescent-shaped excisions at the margin of the hairline; there was no undermining. He observed that "crow's-feet" wrinkling occurs in the form of a triangle, and he deduced that the appropriate correction should be the elevation of the base of the triangle. He followed Passot in relieving the buccolabial sulcus by means of a small preauricular excision, without undermining. For the double chin, he

---

[2]Our translation—as are all others in this chapter—M. G-U.

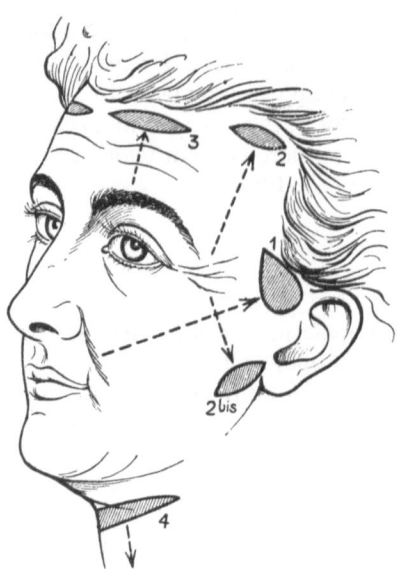

Fig. 2. Passot's skin segment resection technique of 1919, from [98], reproduced with permission

excised a due amount of adipose through an incision following along the submental sulcus. For drooping folds in the cervical region, he made an incision "in the form of a policeman's visor"; the incision started at the rear of the auricular pavilion, curved upward toward the mastoids, and then descended behind them.

In 1920 Adalbert Bettman [8], the first surgeon [106] to publish "before and after" photographs of his procedure, set the precedent for the temporal and preauricular incision used in the contemporary rhytidectomy. It extended well up into the temporal area, contoured the earlobe, and arched upward behind the ear. (A similar incision was described in 1922 by F. A. Booth [9].) Bettman used local anesthetic, a 2% solution of procaine hydrochloride and epinephrine.

Following Miller and Passot, Lagarde [73] was concerned about concealing scarring in frontal and malar area operations; this he did by incising in the hairline. Like them, he estimated the amount of skin to be resected by performing the pinch maneuver in front of the ear.

Bourguet in 1924 [11] was the first to describe hernias of the lower eyelid and the first to prescribe a corrective procedure for them. In 1925 [12] he explained how he came to omit the use of the incision at the level of the zygomatic arch for the correction of the buccolabial fold, incising the scalp instead, after shaving the lower part of the hair in the temporal region.

Bourguet's incision ran parallel to the buccolabial fold, and its length varied with the requirements of the individual patient. He lifted the lower edge of the incision with forceps and detached the entire cheek with scissors, at the same time pulling the skin upward above the upper edge of the incision in order to estimate the degree of elevation of the lower edge of the scalp incision. The necessary amount was excised, and stitching was done with horsehair.

For correction of the scalp, Bourguet described a V-shaped incision beginning behind the earlobe, then running parallel to the retroauricular furrow and

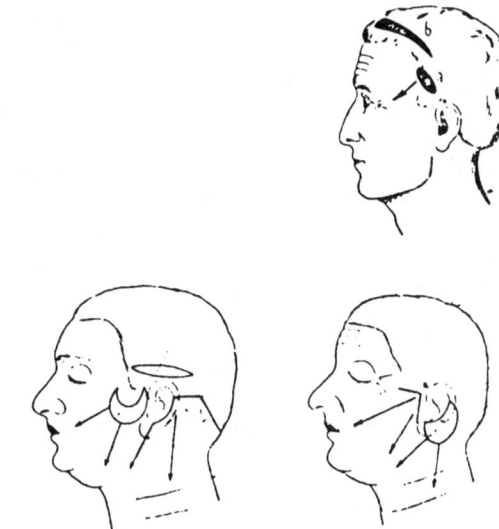

Fig. 3. In 1926 Noël particularly endorsed the use of strategically placed ellipsoidal incisions, Fig. 39–41 from [94], reproduced with permission

descending behind the mastoid, extending through the entire length of the hairline. If there was adherence to the lobe, it was separated with scissors. The flap was detached with the scissors tip to the lower border of the inferior maxillae. As detachment was performed, the cervical skin was pulled upward behind the pavilion. Excess skin was removed, and the suturing was performed.

When the neck and buccolabial fold were undergoing operation simultaneously, the temporal and retroauricular incisions were united by another incision running in front of the helix and on the auditory canal behind the tragus; this prevented folding of the skin. The final sutures were performed over the internal portion of the tragus, thus hiding the scar.

Bourguet's technique for elimination of eyebags consisted of "incising the bottom of the conjunctival bag and expanding the inferior rectus muscle, opening the fibrous bag, then removing the greasy matter [adipose tissue] found in there." He stitched with catgut and positioned other sutures in the conjunctival mucosae.

Noël's book appeared in the medical literature of 1926 [94]. She provided a comprehensive description of surgical procedures for the removal of wrinkles, and she believed it was better to perform two operations that left no discernible traces than to accomplish everything in a single operation leaving scars. Ideal spots recommended for the incision were the hairline and the temporal region.

Before deciding which method of correction to adopt, Noël showed her patient the result that would be obtained. She did this by pulling the patient's skin with metallic forceps covered with rubber, adjusting direction, pattern, and emphasis according to the patient's wishes. Once she had determined the procedure to be used, she made a model of the zone to be resected. In the temporal region the model might have been the shape of an ellipse of varying degrees of eccentricity; of a half-moon, with dissimilar tips; or of an ellipsoidal figure with a curved upper tip and a horizontal lower base. Noël particularly endorsed the ellipsoidal incision (Fig. 3) because its use minimized swelling and necrosis. Noël worked with a view to symmetry by using a "craniometer," and she did not find it necessary to employ anything but a local anesthetic during correction of wrinkling in the temporal area (94). Noël opposed undermining whenever it could produce visible paralysis and hematomas. She stitched by employing single sutures tied by a double knot; if the tension became too strong, she used the Swedish [sic] suture, albeit only a few, since Swedish sutures would leave marks when removed. After 4 days, the sutures on both ends were removed; on the sixth day every other suture was removed, and on the seventh day the remaining sutures were removed.

The Classic Period: Bames, Joseph, Bourguet

The major deficiency of these early techniques was their lack of undermining. This fact was noted in an important paper by Bames [6] in 1927. For permanent results Bames recommended undermining the skin for a short distance. The effect could be enhanced by exploiting the relative inelasticity of the fascia by suturing the flaps of skin onto it rather than over each other. Apparently convinced of prevalent timorousness among his colleagues, Bames acknowledged that his proceudre was "too much for the would-be surgeon," and he reconciled himself to the incorrigibility of his contemporaries in confining themselves to the hairline, "stretching the surrounding skin so tightly that it gives an unnatural, harsh, and drawn appearance to the face."

Bames also stressed the difference between face peeling and the surgical correction of facial wrinkles. He pointed out the distinction between light and deep peeling and emphasized the dangers of facial peeling in contrast to surgery.

In the same year, Stein [118] described a technique for correction of the temporal region. The skin of the scalp was shaved on either side of the temples, and the area to be excised was marked off with typophorobrown [sic]. The amount of skin to be resected was determined during the operation, according to the effect desired, with care taken not to deform the fissura palpebrae. As a second phase of face-lifting, Stein excised two oval or half-moon-shaped pieces of skin on either side under and behind the ear. Sometimes the incision was placed in the scalp at the mastoid to make the scars invisible, though Stein thought this reduced the effectiveness of the operation.

In order not to remove too much skin when removing bags beneath the eyes, Stein determined the limits of excision through frequent closing of the eyelid during the operation. The excisions were mostly half-moon in shape.

For an operation in the retroauricular region, Stein slightly undermined the lower margin of the wound from the bottom in order to gain better tension. Noting that tension at the temple and at the retroauricular and infraorbital fields was ineffectual in removing forehead wrinkles, Stein instead cut out a long, narrow strip of skin behind the hairline of the forehead, parallel to the hairline, and ending on both sides behind the frontal eminence.

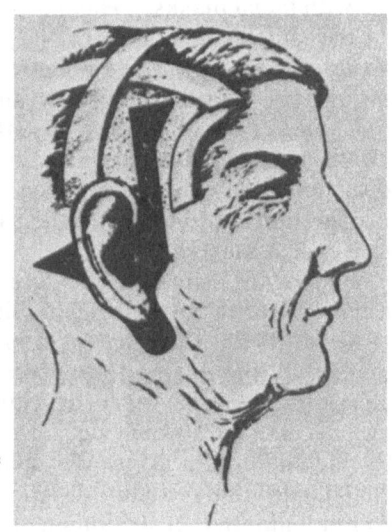

Fig. 4. In Joseph's face-lift operation of 1928, the preauricular incision was modified to closely follow the tragus, thus minimizing visible scarring, from [70], reproduced with permission

As for the double chin, Stein reduced the excess adipose tissue by cutting out a strip of skin along the sagittal plane of the neck, from the chin extremity toward the hyoid. The shape of this skin strip resembled a piece of sliced melon. "The result," he stated, "is a sagittally situated scar that is almost invisible. After healing, it can be removed in the form of a rhomb."

In 1928 Jacques Joseph of Berlin [70] stated that his first operation to correct cheek ptosis was done in 1912. (If correct, this would establish Joseph's claim to priority for that particular operation; but, like a number of other such retrospective assertions, it cannot be independently verified.) "When employing my method at that time," he wrote, "I couldn't avoid a small vertical scar in front of the ear." He explained the modifications he made to eliminate this scar completely, since, while not really noticeable, it was nevertheless visible in front of the tragus as a result of the two linear cuts of his earlier incision. The skin strip removed in front of the tragus left a visible triangular mark after suture. Joseph observed that

> today I make the preauricular rear incision directly at the front border of the antrum auris. Then I remove the skin triangle over the tragus with what remains of the skin strip, and I execute the frontal preauricular incision by saving a corresponding triangle to cover the triangle over the tragus completely, without any external scar after the cheek and throat skin is stretched upward [Fig. 4]. The skin that remains covers the tragus and the skin next to the earlobe. To keep the skin thin and supple, remove the adipose tissue [70].

In 1928 Halla [60] commented on Eitner's claims [32] that "for removal of wrinkles it is necessary to overcorrect" and that, in relation to L-shaped forehead wrinkles, "improvement can already be observed by immobilizing the face with facial masks.'' Halla objected to Eitner's method of stretching (which was the same as Joseph's), on the grounds that it produced visible scars and the danger of injury to the eye oblique muscle and facial nerve. Halla also believed that overcorrection could cause an unnatural distortion of the face, with such broadening of the mouth and nose that another operation would be necessary.

Halla's own face-lifting incision was made a little above and in front of the upper tip of the ear, where he considered it harmless and invisible and where the operation could be repeated as often as needed, provided the skin remained more or less elastic.

He ended his article by mentioning Eitner's failure to mention his own article on removal of facial wrinkles published in 1927 [59].

Also in 1928, Bourguet [13] prescribed a method of correcting forehead wrinkles by paralyzing the nerves responsible for the muscular contractions that are their cause. According to Bourguet's own experience, wrinkles disappear on the paralyzed side. He recommended two methods: 1) injection of an 80% alcohol solution into the facial nerve branches that join frontal muscles which contract involuntarily; this method was not lasting and had to be repeated after 8 months; 2) sectioning of the facial nerve branches of the normal side; the results of this method would be permanent.

Bourguet admitted that both techniques had "minor" drawbacks. Paralysis of both frontal muscles and the subsequent loss of tone would cause these muscles to stretch and the skin to expand, causing the brows to descend and the eyes to appear more deeply sunken in their orbital cavity. To correct this, Bourguet performed a fibrocutaneous or a fibromuscular-cutaneous removal of different magnitudes above the hairline, applying deep surface sutures and shortening the length of the muscle that raises the eyebrows.

For elimination of the buccolabial fold under local anesthesia, Bourguet made an obtuse incision, with its upper border above the zygomatic arch and extending downward and backward. The lower edge circled the line of the pavilion insertion, descending on the edge of the tragus and holding onto its middle part. By a straight incision, both ends of the angle were joined and the circumscribed triangle was separated. He detached the cheek with blunt scissors as near as possible to the buccolabial fold, pulling the skin upward until the lower line of the incision joined the upper one. To avoid quick relaxation due to cutaneous elasticity, he destroyed the elastic fibers by electrocauterization. Then he sutured with horsehair and applied gauze concealed by the hair contours.

If the first portion of the buccolabial furrow could not be corrected, Bourguet suggested placing a grafted section of fat from the same patient under the upper lip. This was inserted below the alae nasi by a sublabial or vestibular incision.

For neck correction having to do exclusively with wrinkles constituting prominences and furrows, Bourguet made a short, crosswise incision under the mental fold or at the height of the hyoid bone, detaching the skin until the lower part of the depression was reached. An autogenous pad of fat was then grafted on. In certain cases, he sectioned the two conspicuous "tendons" (i.e., the inner borders of the platysma) on the inner margin of the cutaneous muscle.

When there was a pendulous pleat in the neck, Bourguet made a cutaneous incision at the front, at the level of the earlobe's connection, and he cut the lobe away if it was attached. He carried the incision toward the mastoidal base, following the retroauricular furrow, and continued downward through the entire length of the hairline, which had already been shaved to a width of approximately 1.5 cm; then the firmly attached skin was dissected on the mastoidal area until the side of the neck was reached, and thence dissection was carried along the full length of the lower maxillary border. Pulling the cervical skin backward obtained the desired tension. Bourguet then removed a portion of skin in the form of "a policeman's cap" (French nationality, circa 1928!), suturing the incision to adjust tension.

For the removal of horizontal forehead wrinkles, Bourguet cut out a long strip of skin parallel to the hairline and closed the wound with a suture. Through the tension of the suture, the forehead skin would stretch upward, eliminating wrinkles. To remove wrinkles at the outer corner of the eye and mouth, he made an excision in the hairy region of the temple and in front of the ear.

In 1929 Schlesinger [108], commenting on a technique described by Kromayer [71], stated that even the most careful technique cannot entirely control the outcome of the scar, since this depends on the patient's healing tendency and on the condition of the skin as well as on the technical prowess of the surgeon. Therefore, Schlesinger thought it better to place the scars where they would not be seen, especially in face-lifting operations, the main purpose of which is to disguise aging. He believed that Kromayer's incision made this impossible, because it crossed the natural line of skin fibers, increasing the chances of scar formation. He did not believe that there was any rule on incisions which could be applied in every case; each case should first be experimented upon to discover direction of stretching, the best one being that which in no way distorted the face. In general, Schlesinger favored Joseph's incision—the excision of a strip in front of the ear and of a triangle above and below the ear.

Schlesinger believed that Kromayer did not take the elasticity of skin into consideration, and this, to him, was the most important and difficult aspect of the operation. Elasticity could stretch the skin like a piece of elastic cloth over the whole face; only then could one see how much and in what location skin should be removed. The flap of skin should then be stitched temporarily until it fit perfectly. For the final suture, Schlesinger suggested using strong catgut threads to fix the flap subcutaneously; this suture was to be done in such a way that the edges of the wound would connect naturally and without tension.

Elaboration of the Early and Classical Techniques

According to Gumpert [58], Noël's disciple, it was essential first to mark out the direction of the incisions and then to follow these strictly, since the appearance of the skin would change irrevocably after injection of the anesthetic.

Lexer [77] stated that the elasticity of the skin dictated both that the wound be undermined and that the flaps of skin not be merely sutured to each other but

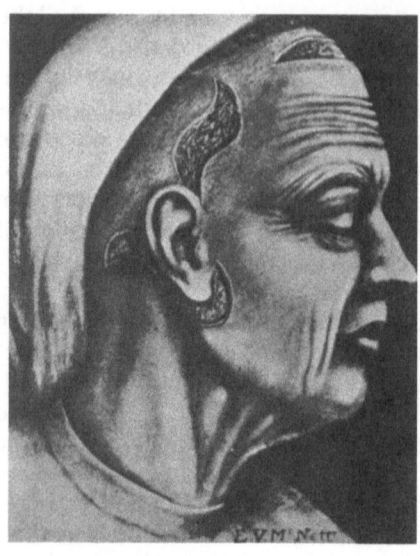

Fig. 5. Lexer's S-shaped incisions (1931) elevated the tissues and avoided the problem of preauricular scarring. (Artist's adaptation of Fig. 1290 in [77], reproduced with permission)

rather fixed to the temporalis fascia. His incisions were in the shape of mirror S's (Fig. 5): One rose vertically from the top of the ear; the other, with a "hook" in front of the lobule, inclined backward at about 45°. Subcutaneous sutures were attached to the periosteum of the mastoid in the region behind the ear.

In 1933 Passot stated what he considered to be the essentials of an operation to counteract facial wrinkling:

the perfect sterility of sutures, avoidance of postoperative edema, ecchymosis, etc., since the patient will recall with delight not only the magnificent outcome but also the ease of the post-operative period, its short duration, and the possibility of keeping the operation a secret [99].

In 1934 Pires [100] described the following method for eliminating wrinkles: after determining the proper size and shape of the skin strip to be removed and then removing it, he performed a deep suture with catgut, connecting the external muscle fibers of the musculus buccinator to the aponeurosis of the temple. He then pulled the skin strip and cut away the excess, suturing the surgical borders with 2-0 thread in the intermediate spaces. Simple healing measures were taken, with removal of sutures after 7-10 days.

In an article written in 1935 [33], Eitner advised caution in accepting patients for rhytidectomy and care in incising at just the proper depth of tissue [33]. For rhytidectomy in the malar region, Eitner used an incision to the depth of the subdermal layer along the preauricular sulcus in front of and above the tragus. Holding this border upward, he cut beneath the area of skin to be excised, precisely at the papillary stratum. Only at this point in the operation was the skin—at the margins where the fragment had been excised—cut more deeply; then stretching the skin upward and suturing it to the layer of the adipose were

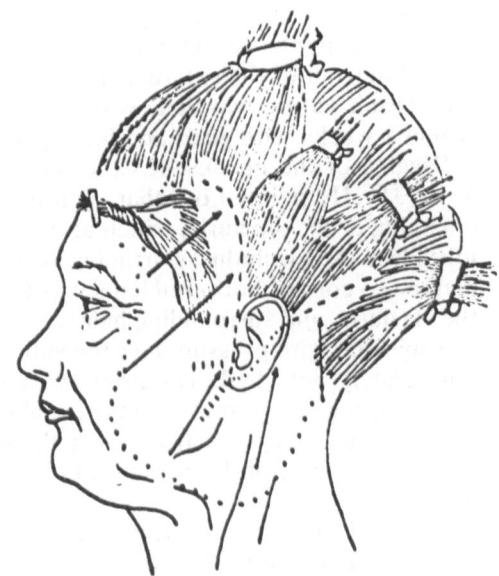

Fig. 6. Burian's contribution of 1936 emphasized the importance of wide undermining if lasting results are to be obtained. Fig. 1 from [19], reproduced with permission

performed. Eitner would supplement the stretching action when it was indicated by undermining to the corner of the patient's mouth.

Like Bames, Burian [19] was an advocate of the thesis that only radical surgery can seriously eliminate the folds that run from the wings of the nose to the mandibulae, drooping of the skin of the throat, and sagging around the eye corners and the orbital arches. He appreciated that added boldness required added preparation and caution. Accordingly, he measured the area to be resected meticulously before the operation, shaved the hair on the operative field, and marked the line of incision in the shaped zone with methyl violet.

As to executing the incision itself, Burian was explicit about the level of dissection: He left about 4 mm of fat attached to the skin. He did not shrink from prescribing wide undermining (Fig. 6):

One must advance toward the cheekbone, where the skin is fixed to the periosteum through rather short and tight retinacula; this definitely must be separated, otherwise it will be impossible to correct the upper part of the buccolabial fold. One then continues down to the corner of the mouth, over the mandibular border, and then to the throat and the sternocleido-mastoideus muscle [19].

In the lower portion of the sternocleidomastoideus, Burian detached the skin at the level of the thin subcutaneous adipose, anticipating modern procedures, and then stretched the skin with clamps, both before and behind the ear. He then marked the strip of excess skin to be cut, suturing at the upper front part of the ear. The hairy skin at the temple region was stretched enough to lift the external part of the orbital arches; then a sickle-shaped piece of skin was excised and this part of the wound sutured immediately with interrupted sutures.

Burian followed the same procedure at the back of the head, suturing around the ear in order to stretch the skin of the "throat." For the visible part of the wound in front of the external ear, suturing was done without any tension; the intradermic suture was done with horsehair. Burian found that the skin healed within 2 weeks with good and lasting results.

Sagging of the cheeks was the focus of Ehrenfeld's operation reported in 1937 [31]. He pointed out that such drooping is "always accompanied by an enlarging of the ala auris, which also sags with an enlarging border." The earlobes lose their roundness, hanging against the facial skin in a shallow line. His method to correct both problems was this: a triangle of hair was shaved above the ala auris, and surrounding hair was fixed with "mastisol." Local anesthetic was injected with pressure into the subcutaneous tissue, and the skin was then immediately detached. The primary incision was made in the temple region. With a strong, deep suture, all the facial skin was pulled up and back, then fixed above the arcus zygomaticus, near the incision and toward the fascia temporalis. The borders of the incision were joined in the incisura auricularis with one or two very fine sutures.

Starting from underneath, the skin was pulled up and back and excised in the line corresponding to the opposite wound border; excision was continued by steps, joining the wound borders with subcutaneous sutures as soon as they were sectioned. If there was excessive skin above the ala auris, Ehrenfeld removed it in a triangular piece. The wound borders were closed with a few fine sutures.

After the hair was cleansed, a small piece of gauze was placed over the wound, and the whole region was covered by hair. The sutures were removed after 4 days. Ehrenfeld noted that "it is useful to apply radiation with a 'Sollux lamp' to the auricular region, to prevent or control possible edema." He stated that his method was uncomplicated, that the scar was nearly invisible, and that there were no facial distortions due to excessive skin excision [31].

By 1944, experience in eradicating wrinkles had accumulated to the point where it was both possible and appropriate to extract some of the principles involved. A few of these were formulated by Cook [25]. In the aging process,

the parts most frequently involved are forehead, neck, mammae, abdomen, thighs, and ankles. . . .Interest in rhytidectomy is not limited to the female alone, the proportions as to sex being about ten females to one male. . . . Rhytidectomy is semimajor surgery, and like all such should only be done in an operating room where the best of surgical technique is available.

The general principle of resection and suture, undermining the skin to be tightened, is the technique employed. In an average case an inch and a quarter, or more, of skin should be excised bilaterally. However, until judgment is acquired by experience, fractional excision should be practiced. The location of the excision depends on where tension is to be exerted [25, pp. 60–62].

In 1948 Galand [43] tersely compressed corrections for many defects into remarkably few words.

Forehead wrinkles. Scalp incision 1 cm away from the forehead skin; frontal detachment; cutaneous abrasion, suture with separated stitches; compressive gauze dressing for four days. Result: unreliable, short-lasting.

"Crow's feet" wrinkles. Diamond-shaped temporal incision on the hair; cutaneous abrasion; suture with separated stitches; compressive gauze; removal stitches after tenth day. Gratifying results for three to four years.

Malar wrinkles. Triangular or diamond-shaped incision, supra- and pre-auricular; deep detachment toward the cheek; compressive gauze dressing for four days; withdraw stitches progressively in ten days. Satisfying results for three to four years.

Hanging cheek and double chin. Pre- and retro-auricular cut; detachment, suture below the separated lobe; compressive gauze four to five days; remove stitches progressively from the sixth to the fifteenth day; apply "carbon snow" on the visible scars. Surpassing results four to five years.

Eyebags. Reduce hernia fat by an incision starting on the external ocular fissure, continuing under the lower eyelashes; compressive gauze for two days; extract stitches on the third day; scarless by the seventh day. Definite and superlative results even when the problem may reappear in four to six years.

Alive to the necessity for concealing scars and preserving a natural post-operative appearance, Brown [16] exploited the earlobe to conceal his incision and to support some of the tension from the temporal area, through excision of a small triangle.

His temporal incision contoured the ear, extending forward in front of the ear and upward into the hairline behind the ear. With the margins of the skin secured with forceps, undermining was prescribed "as extensively as the particular need indicates"; in fact, this translated into a boundary defined by the outer canthus of the eye, the buccolabial fold, and the sternocleidomastoideus. With a view to protection of the facial artery and nerve, the level of undermining was above the fascia. "Anchor" sutures in four areas—the canthus region, the buccolabial fold, along the mandible, and from the sternocleidomastoideus to the postauricular sulcus—preceded resection of the superfluous skin, usually, Brown commented, about 4–5 cm.

Evolution of the Rhytidectomy

With the advent of the 1950s, an increasing number of surgeons gave their attention to the removal of wrinkles. The demand for face-lifts on the part of patients rose sharply, and the elaborations of rhytidectomy multiplied and improved.

In 1950, Mayer and Swanker [85] described their technique for rhytidectomy.[3] They remarked that although the correction for relaxation of the skin of the eyelids was a distinct operative procedure, it was so definitely a part of a complete "rhytidoplasty" that it had to be included in their discussion. They divided their account as follows: cheeks and neck, forehead, upper and lower eyelids.

---

[3]Their term was *rhytidoplasty*.

In the malar region, their incision started 2 cm above the preauricular area and roughly contoured the ear to a point "horizontally opposite the upper limits of the tragus," where it sloped downward 1 cm below the ear. From this line of entrance, undermining at the "superficial subcutaneous level" extended from the lateral canthus of the eye to the buccolabial fold and the oral canthus. The neck was also undermined from the submental region around to the postauricular incision. To keep hemorrhage at a minimum, Mayer and Swanker used scissors in preference to the scalpel. Retention sutures were used to hold the skin at a suitable degree of tension, and the redundant tissue was removed along the lines of the incision.

The line of incision for frontal wrinkles was 1–1.5 cm behind the hairline; it began about 3 cm above the ear and stretched over the forehead. Next, dissection was performed at skin level to the hairline, where it shifted to the adipose tissue level. Generally, it extended as far down as the eyebrows. Then, prior to suturing, the flap was stretched enough to restore the eyebrows to a normal level.

To ameliorate the characteristic drooping of the upper eyelid that takes place with age, Mayer and Swanker selected the first of the folds that occur as the lower margin of a crescent-shaped incision whose upper margin was determined by the amount of skin that could be raised with the forceps. The line of incision in the lower lids started beside the canaliculus orifice about 1 mm below the ciliary border, then moved out along the natural crease at an angle of 45° below the horizontal. The skin was undermined to the level of the orbicularis oris, and herniated infraorbital fat was dissected and removed. Redundant skin was drawn upward and to the side, where the excess was eliminated by section along the upper border and removal of a triangle at the lateral canthus.

In 1952 Seltzer [109] emphasized the importance of performing a very thorough examination of the physical status and the skin condition of elderly patients before undertaking aesthetic surgery. As in the case of Bames [6], the meticulousness of the preliminaries was commensurate with the thoroughness of the operative procedure endorsed. Seltzer considered fastidious care and thoroughgoing operation to be complementary aspects of the rejuvenation process:

> The operation is carried out with all the precautions of major surgery. Anesthetization is of special concern. It has been said that the anesthetic is of less importance than the anesthetist, and this is especially true in operating on older people. . . . From the standpoint of greater permanence of the correction made, an extensive excision is required [109, p 186].

Seltzer's excision followed an integral line stretching from one ear, over the forehead (though only a few centimeters within the hairline), around the ear, then across the occipital hairline. The extensiveness of the incision was matched by the thoroughness of undermining (Fig. 7).

> The success and the degree of permanence of the operation depends in a great degree upon the extent of the undermining of the skin. There is no arbitrary rule for carrying out the undermining, but in general it should depend upon the amount of skin which must be removed, and

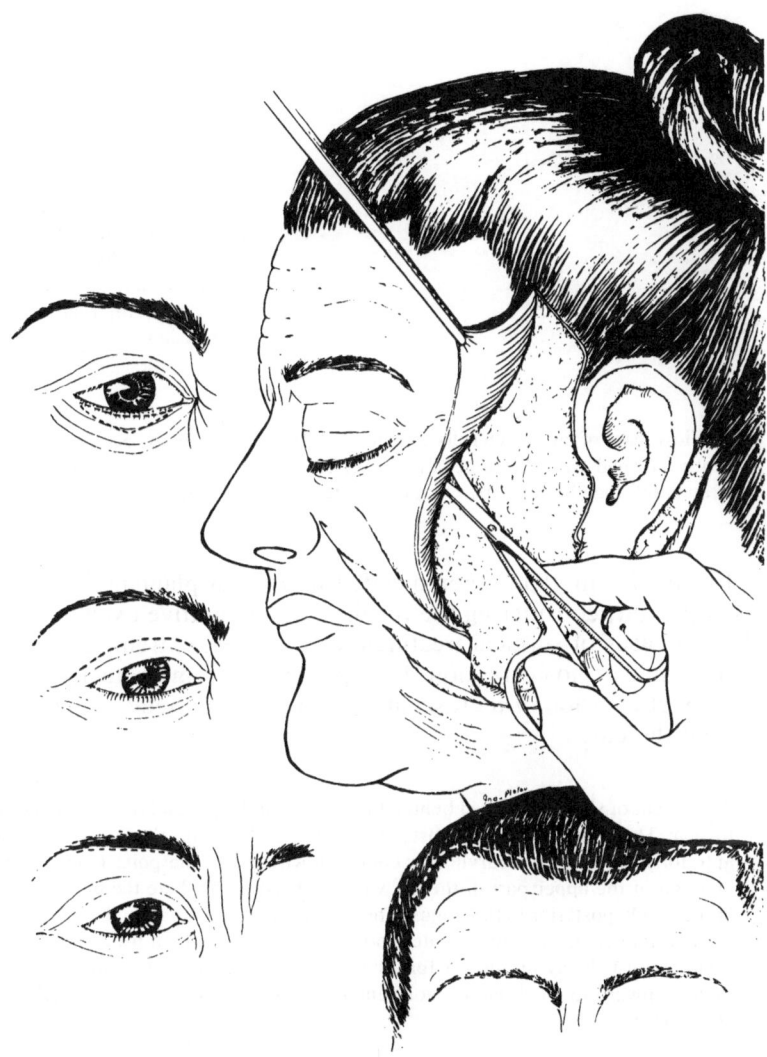

Fig. 7. An extensive incision and thorough undermining were featured in Seltzer's face-lift operation published in 1952. Fig. 1 from [109], reproduced with permission

upon the elasticity of the skin concerned. . . . Since it is well to undermine generously, it should extend nearly to the outer angle of the eye, the edge of the nostril and to the corner of the mouth, care being taken that it is done exactly the same on both sides [109, p 178].

Brown's procedure in 1953 [17] for baggy lower eyelids involved an adaptation for hernia. Following an incision somewhat less precisely defined than Mayer and Swanker's [85], Brown teased the fibers of the orbicularis oris apart, exposing

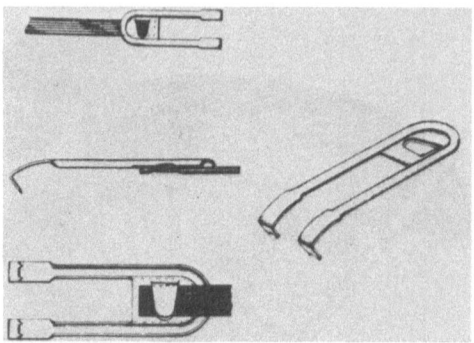

Fig. 8. In 1955 Brown published the details of his prosthesis, which he claimed was easily worn and concealed and obtained the same results as a surgical face-lift. Shown are views of the hairpin-like metal end-piece as seen from above, below, the side, and in perspective. The terminating spicules engage in cloth tabs cemented to the skin. Fig. 1 from [18], reproduced with permission

a yellow mass of fat, which rolls up from the gap in the oribularis oculi muscle. The bulging fat is gently grasped with the forceps and excised with a scissors. We have found that the muscle strands fall together and there is no need to suture them [17, p 187].

Lewis [75] in 1954 recommended individual planning of the procedure for each patient, considering the results of preoperative examinations. He argued that, in cases of surgical treatment of wrinkles, extreme correction may be as undesirable as no correction. His operation to remove facial wrinkles involved the novel excision of a crescent of skin in the parietal region and of a triangle behind the ear.

A crescent of skin is removed behind the hairline in the parietal region and a triangle posterior to the ear. The incision begins almost at the vertex of the scalp, about 4 cm posterior to the hariline anteriorly. It follows a curvilinear course downward to the point immediately in front of the junction of the upper part of the ear with the head. From here the incision extends downward immediately posterior to the tragus. The incision then curves around the lower attachment of the ear and thence upward immediately posterior to the ear; then it turns sharply posteriorly at a point about halfway up the ear for a distance of approximately 5 cm, then sharply downward, thence upward to meet the incision running posteriorly, removing a triangle within the hairline [75, p 337].

Lewis undermined beneath the area of frontal wrinkling at the level of the superficial fascia. If *only* the frontal region was to be corrected, however, Lewis reverted to the early type of correction involving a series of crescent-shaped excisions located slightly above the hairline, with undermining confined to the area immediately surrounding these figures.

Lewis distinguished between two types of bagginess of the lower eyelids: blepharochalasis (described by Fuchs [41, 42]) and ptosis adiposa (described by Sichel [111]), the blepharochalasis, characterized by flaccid eyelid skin, being due to atrophy of the intercellular tissue, and the ptosis adiposa involving atrophy of the tarsoorbital fascia and laxity of the facial bands connecting the eye with the palpebral muscles. Correction of the former condition involved excision of a crescent-shaped strip of skin from the lower eyelid, undermining

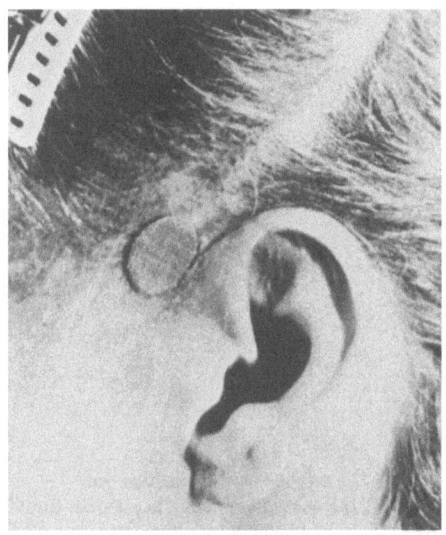 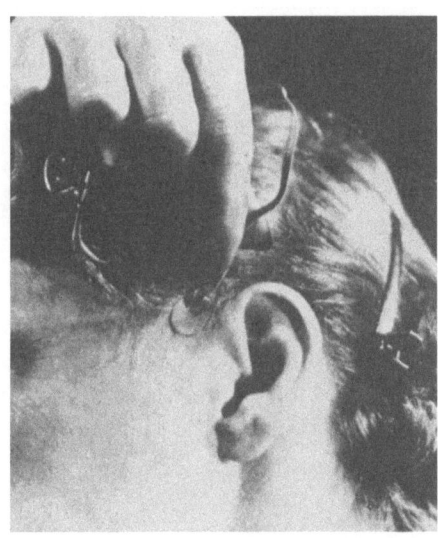

Fig. 9. Cloth tabs of Brown's prosthesis. Fig 2 from [18], reproduced with permission

Fig. 10. Engaging end-piece in cloth tab. Fig. 3 from [18], reproduced with permission

downward for a few millimeters, and resection of a triangle at the outer canthus. For ptosis adiposa, undermining was carried out so that the orbicularis oris was exposed, permitting removal of the herniated fat.

Brendler in 1954 [15] divided the problems of the eyelid into three groups: 1) epiblepharon senile, 2) ptosis adiposa, and 3) blepharochalasis. After dismissing some methods used because of their poor results, for example, massage, compresses, and injections of zinc chloride or paraffin, Brendler declared himself for the use of surgery; but his methods of correcting the upper and lower lids included no significant technique not already described.

In 1955 Johnson [69] recommended that the various rhytidectomy procedures be performed in combinations at the surgeon's discretion. He included the upper eyelids in the first operation. "However," he stated, "the lower eyelids are best done as a separate procedure under local anesthesia." His procedure was like those already described, and it aimed at the same results. In the posterior part of the neck, the incision was placed at the margin of the hairbearing area and extended well down the neck for maximum removal of excess skin.

Johnson warned that incisions inside the tragus were not to be performed, as they frequently deform it. He recommended conservative undermining in the upper cheek and the application of retention sutures at the temporal and mastoid areas.

He removed the submental fat pad through a small incision beneath the symphysis of the mandible. The glabellar furrows were corrected by means of external incision. In the resection of the strip of skin in the lower lid, Johnson instructed his patient to gaze upward while he marked the strip that was to be

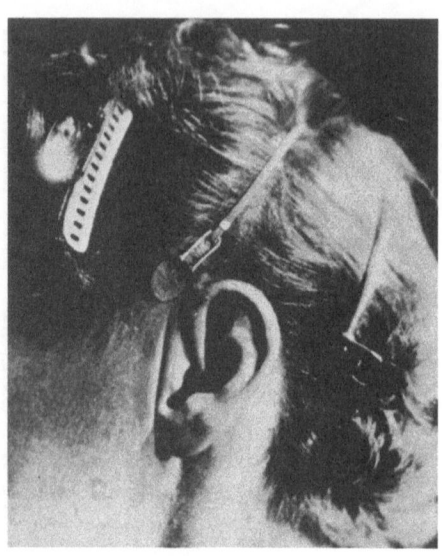

Fig. 11. The prosthesis exerting traction. Combing the hair will conceal the device. Fig. 4 from [18], reproduced with permission

cut out. He then performed a stab opening in the lower lid and placed a suture through it to calculate the amount of skin to be resected. He listed some of the complications of his procedure and the corrections for them:

If a hematoma is suspected at any time it should be evacuated immediately and pressure reapplied. If the hematoma is of any consequence and it recurs, the vessel should be located and ligated.

Slough of a portion of the flap may occur. This may possibly be due to a thin flap, a hematoma, or a combination of both. It may also occur from thrombosis of a vessel in the flap.

In undermining the flaps care must be taken to prevent injury to the facial nerve. Injury to the great auricular, or posterior auricular sometimes occurs causing transitory numbness in the ears or mastoid region [69, p 121].

As a substitute for rhytidectomy, Brown [18] in 1955 described a prosthesis he devised that "can be applied and removed by the patient without aid. Traction is constant and easily concealed by women wearers, and achieves the same effect as a surgical face-lift." Construction and use of the prosthesis (Fig. 8–11) were as follows:

Materials required include a skin film or adhesive composed of polyvinyl butyral, some small oval-shaped fabric tabs of cloth, a length of four-strand rubber elastic covered with cloth, bearing on each end a hairpin-like metal member, each of which terminates with a series of four metal spicules [Fig. 8] designed to engage in the cloth tabs.

In use, each of the cloth tabs is cemented with the polyvinyl butyral adhesive to a position directly in front of and above the ear on a portion of the skin which bears no hair. Into each of these cloth tabs the metal end-pieces of the lifting device are inserted, and the elastic band which stretches across the top of the head can be adjusted to obtain a suitable amount of traction [18, pp 182–183].

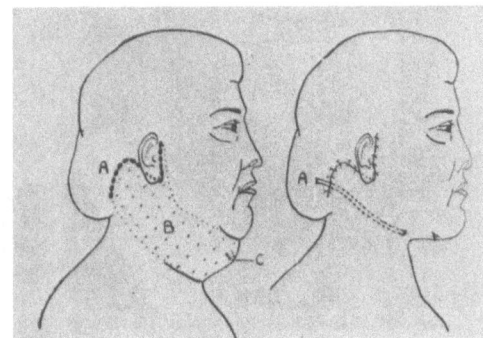

Fig. 12. Spadafora's 1955 operation for suprahyoid adiposity. Fig. 1 from [114], reproduced with permission

The elastic was easily concealed in the hair, and the tabs, when properly applied, could be worn with the confidence that they would not loosen. When in place, the prosthesis comfortably pulled the cheeks into a smooth, youthful contour.

Also in 1955, Davis [28] described a method for what he called "cosmetic meloplasties."

> First, each case should be thoroughly considered. Vanity alone should be critically separated from social or economic factors. Physical factors involved should be carefully weighed. Ability of the patient to withstand the lengthy procedures should govern the surgeon's judgment; also skin texture should be carefully scrutinized. Direction of "pull" should be watched to prevent any displacement of the mouth or eyelids or displacement of the normal hair-bearing areas.

Davis echoed Seltzer [109] in warning that "cosmetic meloplasties" must be given the same preoperative care as any other major procedure. His technical routine was similar to that of his predecessors.

The contribution of Fomon, Bell, and Schattner [37] to the prolific work of 1955 was a set of techniques to avoid the untoward results that accrue when the collagenous fibrils of the skin first contract and then break in advancing age. It was their opinion that, with respect to correcting facial wrinkling, the surgeon must 1) rotate large flaps in front of and behind the auricle and attach them to inelastic fascia; 2) eliminate muscle pull to prevent recurrence of wrinkles, and 3) avoid all tension on the skin to avoid stretching the scar and marginal sloughing of skin. Fomon et al. advised cutting the corrugator and procerus muscles to avoid recurrent glabellar wrinkles and severing the epicranial fibers to avoid forehead wrinkles; both procedures were done through eyebrow incisions. They condemned the use of spindle-shaped excisions of skin to correct wrinkling of the forehead, glabella, neck, and double chin, pointing out that the ephemeral improvement in wrinkling and the development of unsightly scar tissue following this kind of excision had been well demonstrated. For lower eyelid wrinkling Fomon et al. recommended an incision parallel to the lashes and not more than 1 or 2 mm below them, with undermining to the infraorbital

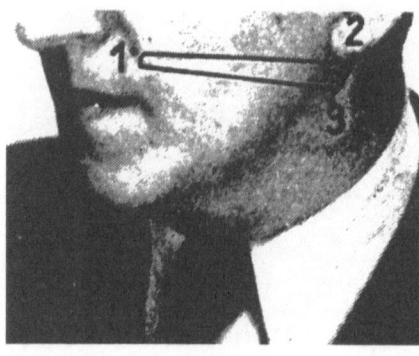

Fig. 13. In 1956 Buttkewitz published his method of elevating tissues by means of subcutaneously applied nylon thread. Shown is the correction for drooping buccolabial fold. Fig. 3 from [20], reproduced with permission

rim and rotation of the skin flap outward and upward [37]. The resultant scar was concealed by the cilia.

Spadafora [114] reported on suprahyoid fat in 1955, which he removed in a manner similar to that of Bourguet [11-14]. In patients with double chin with increase of the transverse diameter of the neck, the problem was corrected by means of a lower malar and cervical rhytidectomy; wide undermining was carried out toward the center of the neck, where it connected with the suprahyoid tunnel, from which adipose tissue was removed through a submental incision (Fig. 12). In patients with thick sternocleidomastoid muscles, Spadafora removed a whole-width slice. He carefully avoided the upper and deeper part of these muscles lest the spinal nerve be damaged or the functioning of the muscle impaired.

In 1956 Buttkewitz [20] proposed a method of eliminating facial wrinkles that did not involve excision of strips of skin and hence obviated the scars left by such excisions. Tissue stretching was carried out subcutaneously with synthetic surgical suture material placed and maneuvered with the help of specially designed needles. Buttkewitz's correction exploited the fact that many faces, particularly those of women, owe their aging appearance to the presence of various types of protuberances, and that these protuberances may be easily removed by subcutaneously applied nylon thread slightly stretched. The technique was simple. With the specially designed needles the thread was introduced directly into the protuberance—for example, in the buccolabial fold—and was fixed under the skin (Fig. 13). The only subsequently discernible signs of this procedure were the minute needle punctures.

For ptosis of the cheeks, a point of suspension was chosen at the hairline near the temple. Buttkewitz said his method was effective for wrinkles of the neck, provided these were not inordinately extensive and deep [20]. If they were not, they could be eliminated by transfixing them laterally; if they were, more traditional methods had to be used. Horizontal forehead wrinkles could be adjusted by means of a nylon thread placed vertically from the wrinkle or by pulling the thread in an oblique direction. Wrinkles between the eyes could be easily removed by a thick bundle of threads placed subcutaneously to upholster the skin and adjust it. This method could not be used to correct excess skin on the upper or lower lid—here the customary means were necessary—nor could

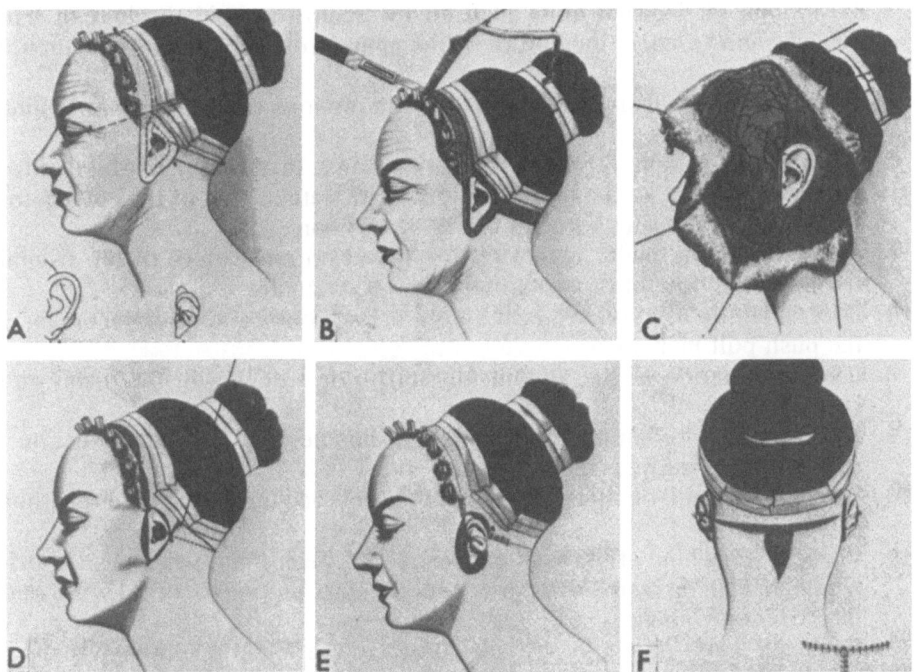

Fig. 14. González-Ulloa's "ear-island" rhytidectomy of 1956. **A** Tracing of lines of incision. **B** Incision begun. **C** Wide detachment of skin around the ear. **D** Stretching of the skin. **E, F** Lateral and posterior views, showing direction of sutures. Fig. 1 from [45], reproduced with permission

fine wrinkles normally be eliminated by Buttkewitz's nylon thread technique. He employed local anesthesia and No. 3 or 6 nylon thread.

To the Present Day

The "ear-island method" of González-Ulloa published in 1956 [45] was the predecessor to contemporary procedures for correction of total facial wrinkling. It had the following advantages: 1) uniform peripheral tension, 2) adequate stretching of all areas of descent of the fact, 3) restoration of facial skin to its original pregravitational position, 4) inclusion in the correction of the entire expanse of the neck, and 5) greater duration of the operative benefits.

The ear-island procedure involved a number of deviations from preceding techniques (Fig. 14), including the following:

1. Continuity of the band of resection from the center of the head to the center of the neck
2. Resection of compensating triangles in the center of the head and neck to equalize the length of both skin margins, thus avoiding pleats and so-called dog-ears and aiding in the antigravitational effect of the procedure and in the accurate suture of the wound

61

3. Positioning of incision quite high on the scalp to avoid the loss of hair follicles and to allow the suture of the aponeurosis epicranialis to anchor the flap
4. Placing the nape incision high to avoid an obvious transverse scar behind the ear
5. Undermining of the forehead extending down to the upper orbital ridge and, if necessary, to the tip of the nose, with detachment of the corrugator and procerus muscles through the same incision
6. Elevation of the malar region by the resection and suture of the frontal triangle; this base often being more than 6 cm wide
7. Determination of tissues to be resected in the frontal and occipital areas by the push-pull maneuver
8. Predetermination of the amount of skin to be resected in the malar and cervical areas
9. Meticulous undermining of the malar area and neck by "tunnel dissection" to avoid severing vessels or nerves
10. Symmetry of pull obtained by two pilot lines traced from the outer canthus of the eye
11. Vertical stretching of the total expanse of the neck (both vertical and horizontal) produced by the resection, undermining, and suture of the band and the occipital triangle
12. Extensive undermining of the neck down to the fossetta supraexternalis
13. Purse-string suture to isolate the ear from the operative field

In 1957 Malbec [83] described his operation for rhytidectomy in full detail. Using a method not greatly different from those described above, he sectioned the aponeurosis without damaging it. His incision contoured the auricular lobule, following the retroauricular sulcus, and after extending 5–7 cm, ran on obliquely until it touched the center of the opposite side. Malbec undermined widely with curved, blunt scissors, reaching the angle of the eye and detaching all the muscular adhesions of this area to remove the crow's-feet. He tried to make a dissection without sectioning the vascular connection from the bottom to the lower border of the skin. Sometimes he used his index finger enveloped with gauze to obtain a wide, easy undermining.

Malbec evaluated the degree of skin to be resected according to the patient's sex, the presence or absence of adipose tissue, and the thinning of the skin that may have occurred with age. Using Chaput's forceps, he picked up the skin rim throughout its contour and, with a slight traction toward the opposite direction, calculated the line of the resection and marked the reference points in order not to have to speculate while operating. It was his view that for a successful outcome, the most significant resection was one performed in the frontal-parietal region as well as in the mastoid-occipital area, where the correcting lines of tension should be placed. To estimate the amount of skin to be resected, Malbec recommended traction on the anterior flap while the assistant was pushing the posterior flap. He stressed carrying out meticulous hemostasis, avoiding tension on the earlobe when suturing, and applying an adequate compressive dressing and bandage.

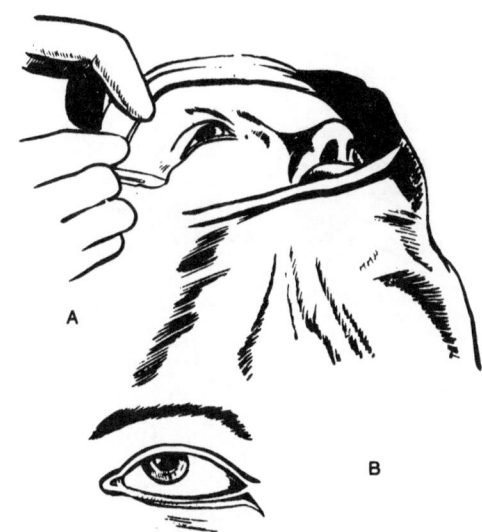

Fig. 15. Hollander's lower lid operation of 1958. A The lateral aspect of the incision beneath the lower tarsus of the right eye. B A similar incision on the left eye shows the excised tissue. Fig. 1 from [66], reproduced with permission

In the same year, 1957, M. M. Hollander [67] described his operative technique for cheek and neck wrinkles. A distinctive feature of this technique was passing the incision along the superior posterior surface of the tragus, after which it was brought interiorly once more, passing around and under the attachment of the earlobe. Hollander also brought the posterior incision along the posterior insertion of the ear and then, at a point just two-thirds above the base of the auricle, he brought the incision posteriorly to the hairline; he entered the hairline and then carried the incision along a downward-curving arch that extended for about 4 cm, depending on the amount of excess tissue present in the neck.

At the initial point above the ear the incision was extended anteriorly for about 1 cm perpendicular to the original incision. Hollander applied three or four subcutaneous supporting sutures, inserting them according to the marks drawn on the skin before the operation; he attached the anterior flap to the temporal fascia and anchored the posterior one in the occipital fascia. The sutures were placed beneath the undermined flaps so that they gave support to the orbicularis oris, the triangularis, the risorius, and the zygomaticus muscles, as well as to the superficial portion of the masseter and the platysma.

When Hollander trimmed the skin in front of the ear, he did so around the tragus, forming a "snug" cover for the cartilage. He continued trimming around the bottom portion of the ear, placing another suture behind the lobule about 1.5 cm up from the point of attachment of the lobe.

Hollander avoided the dog-ear of skin at the initial point of incision above the ear by cutting away the excess skin. Thus he was practically employing the method currently used, in which two triangles are cut, one anterior and one posterior, the former elevating the cheek and the latter the neck.

Hollander's procedures for ameliorating wrinkling of the forehead and of the eyes were outlined in his paper of 1958 [66]. Like Lewis [75], Hollander distin-

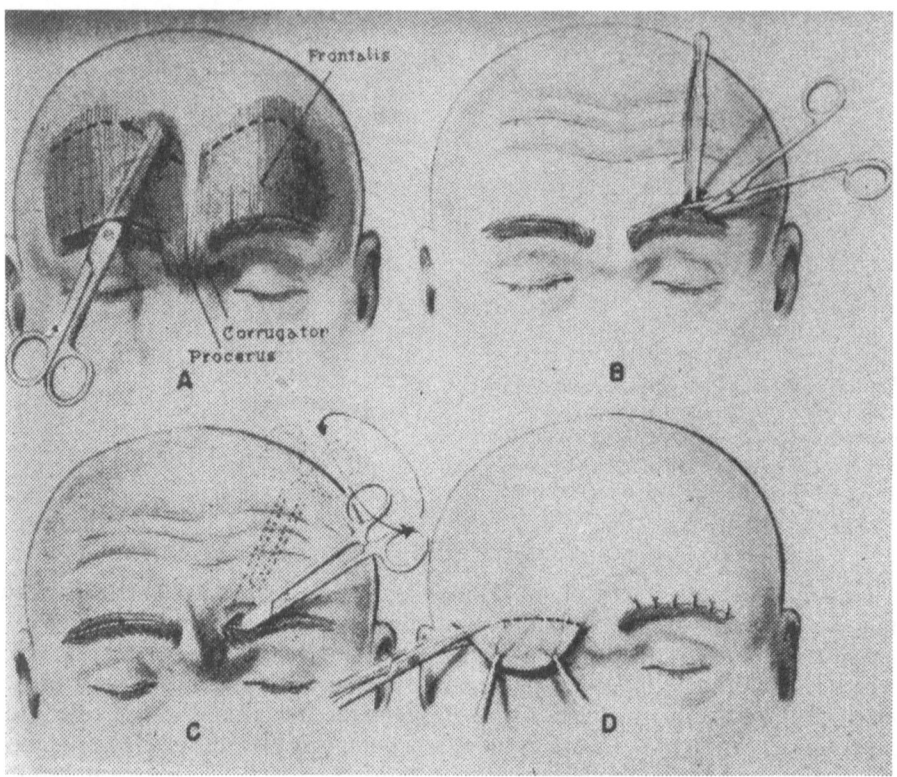

Fig. 16. In 1961 Fomon et al. advocated eliminating the pull of the corrugator, procerus, frontalis, and orbicularis muscles to eradicate forehead wrinkles. This was done by dissecting free or avulsing the muscular insertions and by destroying the frontal branch of the facial nerve. Fig. 8 from [38], reproduced with permission

guished between blepharochalasis and ptosis adiposa, neither of which, again, were considered identical with simple herniation of fat, which is primarily a problem of the adipose content of the orbit. Hollander felt that the lower lid presented the more elaborate problems, which were to be approached by way of a crescent-shaped incision beneath the lid, turned diagonally downward at a 45° angle into one of the wrinkle lines radiating from the canthus. After undermining, the area was examined to determine whether the problem was primarily one of redundant skin or one of fat herniated through the orbital fascia. If there was herniated fat, it was removed and the fascia was sutured. If there was redundant skin, it was removed in the manner shown in Figure 15. To correct wrinkling of the forehead, Hollander joined the growing number of surgeons who used an incision behind the hairline, stretching from one temple to the other, as a preliminary to extensive undermining down to the level of the eyebrows.

By 1961, Fomon et al. [38] had developed new points of view extending beyond their primarily evaluative position of 1955 [37]. They divided the re-

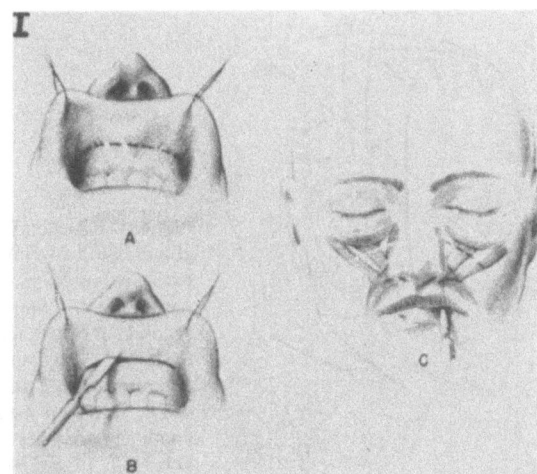

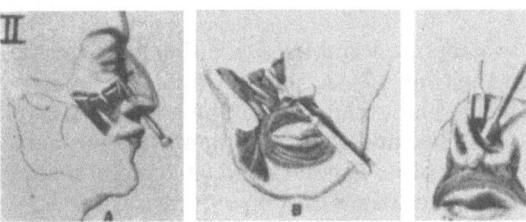

Fig. 17. Fomon et al. also recommended destruction of the quadratus labii superioris to eliminate wrinkles generated by the buccolabial sulcus. The quadratus superioris may be reached by oral or nasal routs. Fig. 11 from [37], reproduced with permission.

quirements of a successful face-lift into two classes: removal of excess skin and eradication of wrinkles. They considered the standard rhytidectomy adequate to meet the first requirement but inadequate to meet the second. To supplement the excision of surplus tegument, they believed curtailment of the action of the mimetic muscles of the forehead, glabella, buccolabial region, and around the mouth, chin, and neck was indicated, since these muscles of expression are quite as fully responsible for wrinkling as the reduction of adipose volume and the loosening of the skin.

To ameliorate wrinkling of the forehead and upper face, they recommended destroying various muscular elements along with the branches of the facial nerve that serve them. Access to the corrugator, procerus, frontalis, and orbicularis muscles was through an incision made along the eyebrow (Fig. 16). Blunt scissors served to separate the skin from the underlying structures. Before the muscles were dissected free, the supraorbital vessels and nerves were identified; following dissection, the muscles were held with a forceps and shortened by about 1 cm. Destruction of the procerus and frontalis muscles was by avulsion with a hemostat. The frontal branch of the facial nerve was destroyed beneath the 1-cm-square section of the frontalis muscle at a point 2.5 cm above and 2.5 cm to the side of the outer canthus.

In the middle of the face, the muscle primarily responsible for the buccolabial sulcus is the quadratus labii superioris. Its action is instrumental in the expression of grief, contempt, defiance, and pain. The approach to curtail its pow-

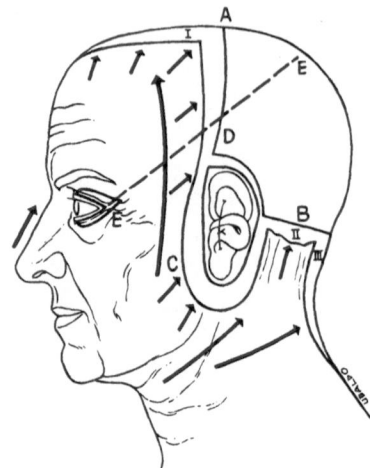

Fig. 18. González-Ulloa's 1962 operation for the integral elimination of wrinkles, using traction triangles and extensive undermining. The first triangle (I) was traced with its vertex on the middle line of the frontal region. The second set of triangles (II) consisted of a pair with the base at the retroauricular region and the vertex toward the posterior medial line. The third triangle (III) was placed on the posterior medial line and lengthened downward as much as necessary to obtain good lifting of the cervical skin. Fig. 1 from [46], reproduced with permission

er to generate wrinkles was either through the oral cavity or through the nasal passage (Fig. 17). A sharp periosteal elevator was used to explore for a line of cleavage below the fascia. The elevator was placed over the frontal process of the maxilla, and then the quadratus was removed by curet against the bone, disposing of its angular head. Its orbital and zygomatic heads were disposed of in the same way.

The principal culprit in wrinkling of the lower part of the face is the quadratus labii inferioris. Fomon et al. recommended intraoral or extraoral approaches as equally effective in immobilizing its wrinkling activity, provided all incisions were kept carefully within a node of muscle fibers (the "Knoten of Eisler") marking the decussation of fibers controlling the oral commissures. A section 1 cm wide was removed from the complex of quadratus, triangularis, and mentalis muscles.

In the neck, fibrosis of the platysma muscle contributes importantly to cervical wrinkling. It was dissected in two flaps: the anterior flap with a blunt dissector, and the posterior flap with a sharp dissector. As the main offset to wrinkling involved rotation of these flaps (with hemostats), the extent of undermining was determined by the amount of rotation required, which was tested empirically during the intervention by attaching the flaps to the margin of the incision with two or three small clamps.

In 1961 Erich [34] described a rhytidectomy[4] technique quite similar to Hollander's [67]. Erich, however, advised carrying the undermining only so far as an imaginary vertical line passing through the outer canthus of the eye (occasionally more extensive undermining would be in order). He recommended that the undermined skin flaps be drawn backward over the ear until enough tension was generated to obliterate wrinkles and unnatural folds of skin, but he emphasized that one should not draw the skin flap upward or downward, because this may well produce an undesirable elevation or descent of the skin.

---

[4]Erich preferred the term "rhytidoplasty" [34].

Pangman and Wallace [97] made the rhytidectomy incision in much the same way as their predecessors did, deviating only in the temporal area, where it was carried down to include the superficial fascia to facilitate dissection. This was mostly done with the fingertip, to cause less bleeding and to provide fair fixation into the deep temporal fascia in the lifted position. Thus a good lift was facilitated with minimal skin removal and without tightening the rest of the scar. Pangman and Wallace reported that the scar left by this procedure was quite satisfactorily unobtrusive.

The superficial and the deep fascia of the temporal regions are fused just above the zygomatic arch. For an effective face-lift, Pangman and Wallace advised sectioning the skin along this line [97]. Dissection was kept superior and superficial to the motor nerves running to the eyelids, its extent varying from case to case. When the neck was involved, undermining was carried across the midline and continued down across the throat and neck. Excess fat was removed from the neck with a curet or scissors or both. In the first step of repair, the fascia above the zygomatic arch was sutured to the deep temporal fascia with a row of interrupted 3-0 sutures. The cheek was lifted, as the fibrous tissue was picked up and plicated with similar sutures. The line of plicating sutures was placed either on the malar eminence or inferior to it, and it extended downward in front of the ear, occasionally including tissues of the neck. Plicating was done at the exact position on the opposite side. The skin was tailored in the usual manner, and drainage was applied. Six weeks after the rhytidectomy, Pangman and Wallace advised dermabrasion combined with a phenol peel of the lids [97]. Routine plastic surgery of the eyelids was performed after the face-lift.

Pangman and Wallace treated deep forehead lines and low eyebrows by extending the rhytidectomy incision across the forehead, either along the hair margin or about 1 cm above the hairline. The skin was elevated from the underlying tissues and pulled back, the excess skin removed, and the wound closed. As for the frown, a small incision was made on the medial end of each eybrow. The skin was elevated away from the corrugator muscle, which was severed along a line curving upward and medially from the eyebrow incision, but only a segment of muscle in the area between eyebrow and nose was removed. The incisions were sutured with fine silk, and a pressure dressing was applied.

The same workers described another way to eliminate frown and forehead wrinkles: the motor nerves supplying the area could be severed [97]. To achieve lift of the eyebrows if this was done, it was necessary to remove a crescent of skin above the superciliary arch.

In 1962 González-Ulloa [46] presented a technique for integral elimination of facial wrinkles that involved careful preoperative tracing, the use of traction triangles, and extensive undermining. Preoperative tracing ran vertically from one temporal region to the other (line A, Fig. 18). It crossed the cranium well behind the hairline; then it curved forward, continued along the preauricular sulcus, and followed the lower portion of the lobule. Continuing at 5-6 mm from the retroauricular sulcus, the trace thus described a circle around the pinna and joined the temporal incision. Isolation of the ear in this way made possible an integral peripheral pull on the whole facial skin.

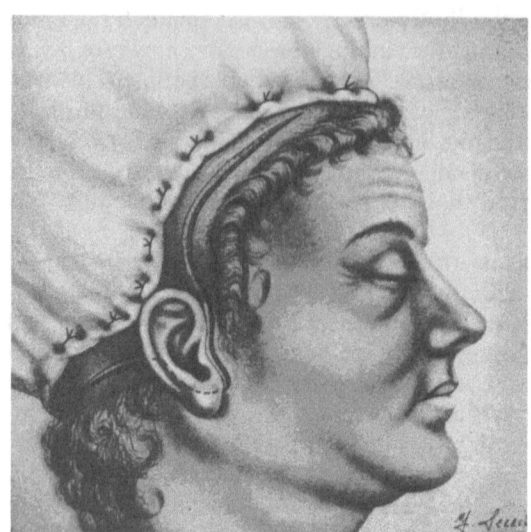

Fig. 19. Fischer's rhytidectomy incision of 1963. Fig. 1 from [36], reproduced with permission

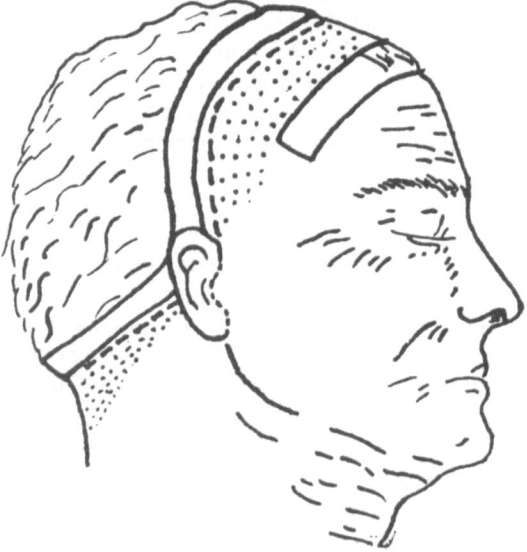

Fig. 20. Farina's rhytidectomy incision of 1964. Fig. 1 from [35], reproduced with permission

The occipital line was next to be traced, starting in the retroauricular region from a virtual prolongation of the lower ridge of the auricular fossette, which served as a reference point for initiating the trace (line B, Fig. 18). It continued toward the posterior midline, where it met with its opposite. The amount of skin to be excised from in front of and below the ear was determined by pinching in the auricular region and then tracing a second line parallel to the first (line C, Fig. 18). The width of the tracing decreased in the temporal region, the area of maximum tension (line D, Fig. 18).

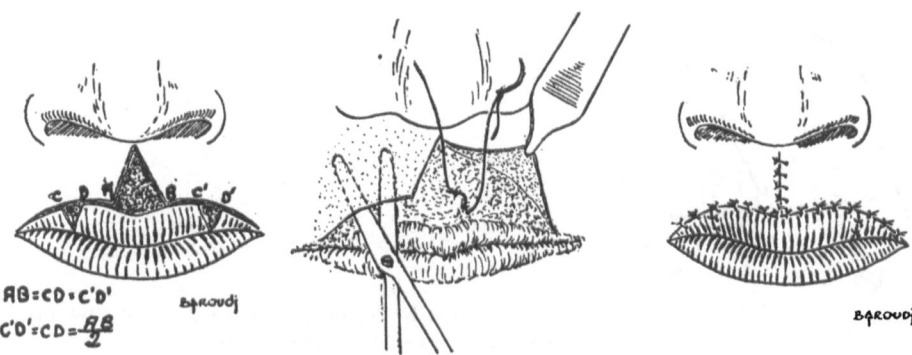

Fig. 21. Farina's correction for the wrinkled upper lip. After incision along the border, a single stitch in the muscular connective tissue would elevate the lip and enhance its fullness. Fig. 3. from [35], reproduced with permission

To achieve antigravitational traction, three sets of triangles were resected. One triangle, lifting the cheeks and the frame of the lids, had its vertex on the midline of the frontal region; its base was twice the width of the strip of skin to be resected beneath the lobule of the ear. The second set of triangles consisted of a pair with the base at the retroauricular region and with the vertex toward the posterior medial line. The third triangle was situated on the posterior medial line at the nape of the neck; its base was on the occipital line and its vertex below it. Excision of this and of the two retroauricular triangles provided strong antigravitational tension in both the cervical and submandibular areas.

After incision and resection of the frontal triangle, undermining, as extensive as needed to provide the amount of lift desired, was carried out. In the lateral part of the neck, undermining was done first, after which the base of the retroauricular triangles was determined by stretching the skin upward and outward.

González-Ulloa emphasized that to provide adequate lift, sufficient undermining must be performed, and that in performing adequate undermining, knowledge of the subcutaneous layers was imperative to avoid damage to the small branches of the facial nerve in the temporal region. These nerve branches were protected by transferring the depth of undermining from the supraperiosteum in the forehead to a supraaponeurotic layer in the temporal region.

The procedure of Krushinski and Pakovich, published in 1962 [72] involved no major departures from that of Pangman and Wallace [96]. Baker [2] and Litton [78, 79] prescribed auxiliary face-peeling procedures—they called them chemosurgery—to be carried out concurrently with rhytidectomy.

In 1963 Marino [84] proposed again a strategy based on a technique derived from that of McIndoe of surgically curtailing the action of the frontal muscle for permanent amelioration of forehead wrinkling. The musculocutaneous flap was dissected at the adipose tissue layer, cutting downward until the frontal and corrugator muscles were disinserted. Marino stressed that the vascular and nerve-carrying pedicles serving the flap should not be severed; this was achieved by dissection of a vascular lamina, the "mesotemporalis," containing

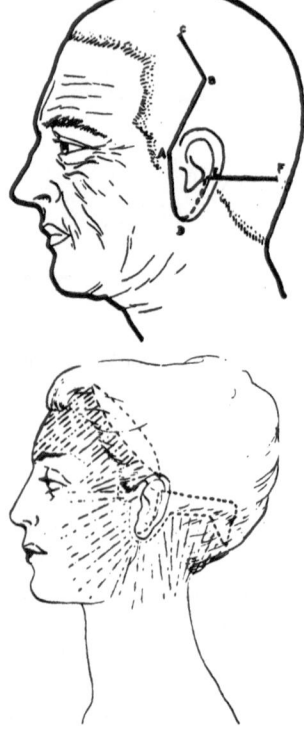

Fig. 22. Serson-Neto's rhytidectomy incision of 1964. Fig. 3 from [110], reproduced with permission

Fig. 23. Talamás placed her rhytidectomy incision just outside the hairline. Fig. 1 from [120], reproduced with permission

the frontal branches of the facial nerve and anterior branch of the temporal artery. After dissection of the frontal flap and of the mesotemporalis, the skin to be removed was marked; and with delicate instruments, the deep layer of the frontal muscle and the necessary parts of the corrugator were resected. Surplus teguments were sectioned, and sutures were placed without drainage.

Fischer's incision of 1963 [36], similar to that of the pioneers of rhytidectomy, was placed inside the hairline to correct wrinkling of the forehead, face, and neck (Fig. 19). Neuernbergk's incision, reported in 1963 [93], was made between the temple and the neck within the hairline, in a preauricular location behind the tragus and in a postauricular location in the fold of the ear. At the temple region, the incision turned at a right angle if the hair was thin; with fuller hair or looser skin or both, it curved in the form of a bow. The incision behind the ear extended to the upper ear, then made a 90° turn. It ended thus in the shape of an inverted bow. Throughout, it was kept within the hairline down through the neck and, as far as possible, to the linea nuchae.

Neuernbergk undermined to the external angle of the eyelid, to the angle of the mouth, and toward the neck at least 12 cm from the root of the ear along the sternocleidomastoideus. The detached skin, pulled over the ear, was fixed with catgut, first behind the auricle at the hairline and then in front of the auricle at the upper ear. The triangles of skin thus formed were excised; depending on their position, the incision could be either bow-shaped or rectilinear.

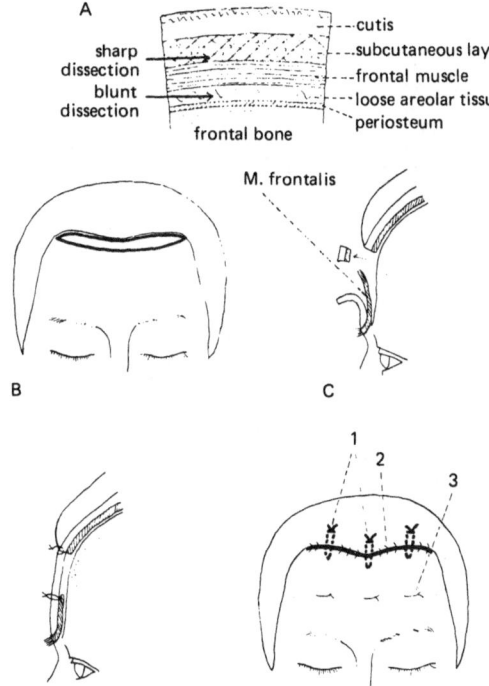

Fig. 24. Uchida's 1955 operation for the correction of frontal wrinkling. **A** Cross section of frontal soft tissues. **B** Incision of frontal muscle. **C** Cross-section view after dissection. **D** The relocated insertion of the frontal muscle and closure of the superficial layers. **E** The mattress sutures **(1)** in position; **(2)** dermal sutures; **(3)** mattress sutures for the frontal muscle. Fig. 2–5 from [123], reproduced with permission

Edgerton et al. [30], in 1964, reported favorably on the use of the peripheral rhytidectomy [45]. They found it advisable to shorten the facial muscles and to pleat the parotid fascia for deep-layer support.

Farina [35] also performed a peripheral incision 2–3 cm from the hairline (Fig. 20). To correct wrinkles of the lip, an incision along the border of the upper lip was recommended. A single stitch was placed in the muscular connective tissue to accent the elevation and enhance the fullness of the upper lip (Fig. 21).

Serson-Neto [110] defined three basic principles of rhytidectomy: 1) traction and sliding of the undermined skin of the face perpendicular to the wrinkles; 2) excision of excess skin; and 3) placement of scar-bearing incisions in hidden areas such as the scalp and the retroauricular region. Serson-Neto's own incision started at the temporauricular point of insertion (Fig. 22, **A**), pursued a posterosuperior course until it reached the parietal prominence (Fig. 22, **B**), then turned and continued for 4–5 cm with a medial upper course (Fig. 22, **C**). The inital incision descended vertically along the juxtaauricular region (Fig. 22, **D**) and around the earlobe. It continued to the middle of the posterior part of the auricle (Fig. 22, **E**), then ran horizontally to the occipital region (Fig. 22, **F**).

Talamás [120] preferred to place the incision outside the hairline, leaving a scar that she claimed was barely visible (Fig. 23). For correction of double chin she made a small incision along the natural line that almost always exists beneath it; the length of the incision was not to exceed 4–5 cm if it were not to be

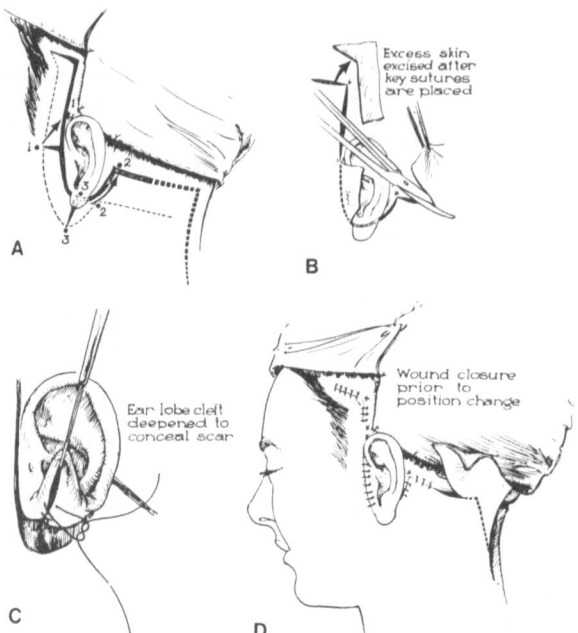

Fig. 25. Spira, Gerow, and Hardy's cervicofacial rhytidectomy. The posterior line extended into the suboccipital region. Fig. 4 from [116], reproduced with permission

noticed. She then detached the skin from the entire area until juncture was made with the temporal incision. All redundant adipose was removed.

In 1965 Uchida [123], cutting immediately below the hairline (Fig. 24), dissected the frontalis muscle en bloc from the subdermal layers and periosteum of the wrinkled area and lowered its insertion from the galea aponeurotica to a point in the middle of the frontal area; thus the wrinkle-making action of the frontal muscle was significantly curtailed.

Skin thickness as a factor in aging and in the duration of rhytidectomy was the subject of a report published by González-Ulloa and Stevens in 1965 [52]. This report also examined the structural changes that accompany facial aging.

In 1967 González-Ulloa, Stevens, Loewe, de la Cruz, and Noble [55] reported on the use of dimethylpolysiloxane (360 Medical Fluid prepared by the Dow Corning Center for Medical Research) as an adjunct to rhytidectomy. Perfusion of dimethylpolysiloxane was claimed to be a chemically innocuous and aesthetically serviceable means of restoring volume lost by the gradual absorption of adipose tissue in the face.

Spira, Gerow, and Hardy [116] reported in 1967 a cervicofacial rhytidectomy based on the classic type of incision in front of and back of the ear, but they extended it posteriorly, and at the root of the helix the line was carried into the suboccipital region (Fig. 25). In rhytidectomy for the male, the skin incision extended along the sideburn up into the temple, just within the hairline. Dissection was carried anteriorly—undermining the temple and the cheek to the malar eminence—and inferiorly to the buccolabial fold, along the corner of the mouth and down the neck. Over the mastoid process, where the ster-

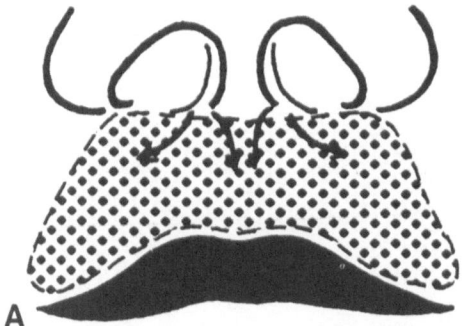
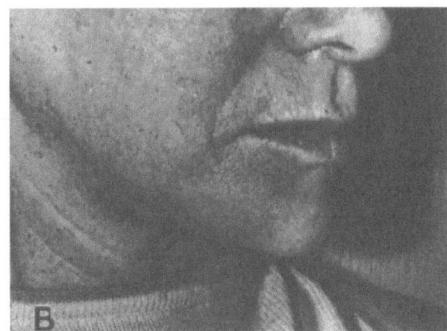
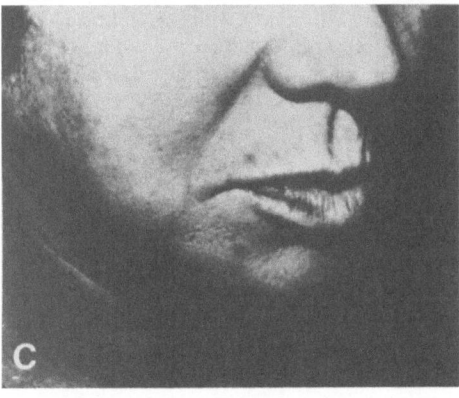

Fig. 26. In 1970 Hinderer reported his correction of deep wrinkles of the upper lip through temporary implantation of a thin Silastic sheet. **A, B, C** Preoperative and postoperative views. Fig. 19 from [64], reproduced with permission

nocleidomastoideus muscle is partially inserted into the skin, dissection was sharp.

The correction for double chin presented by Millard, Pigott, and Hedo in 1968 [88] began with a horizontal incision in the submental crease to a depth of 2-3 cm. The skin of the submental area was dissected from the adipose pad down to the level of the thyroid cartilage with long, blunt scissors. Care was taken to leave a cushion of fat on the lower surface of the skin; and the fatty pad was dissected off the muscle for as far as one could clearly and safely see. Any outstanding vertical bands of the platysma were divided in midarch, well away from all branches of the facial nerve.

Simultaneous performance of peripheral rhytidectomy, blepharoplasty, and adipose tissue restitution with dimethylpolysiloxane was described by González-Ulloa and Stevens in 1968 [53]. The incisions on the upper and lower lids collectively were in the form of an almond, permitting removal of excess fat and excess skin in the vicinity of the outer canthus and facilitating the pulling of the external commissure of the lids upward and outward, as in the young eye.

In another paper delivered in 1968 [54], González-Ulloa and Stevens proposed two styles of rhytidectomy for men. When the results desired were conservative, an incision with the shape of a Roman U was to run from the temporal region; this made possible the resection of two triangles—one preauricular

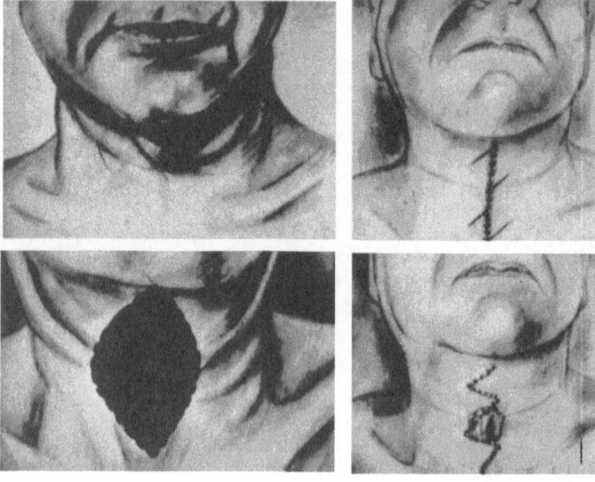

Fig. 27. Carlin and Gurdin's correction of turkey-gobbler neck with ellipse incision and Z-plasty closure. Fig. 4 from [24], reproduced with permission

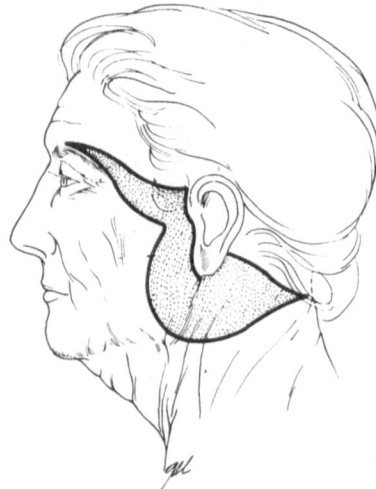

Fig. 28. Carlin and Gurdin's brow lift and rhytidoplasty. Fig. 6 from [24], reproduced with permission

and the other retroauricular—of a base as wide as required for proper stretching.

When a more thoroughgoing rejuvenation effect was in order, González-Ulloa placed the incision around the ear. Its line followed that of the preauricular sulcus and sloped down behind the insertion of the ear at a distance of 5 mm. A second trace was made in front of and beneath the ear at a distance calculated by pinching at the desired tension. These peripheral incisions were joined by a transverse line in the occipital region running from a virtual prolongation of the lower ridge of the triangular fossetta of the antihelix. Undermining extended to the orbital ridge and the malar and cervical areas. A centrifugal pull removed the wrinkles of both the face and the neck.

Baker and Gordon in 1969 [3] warned that the flap left by incising in front of

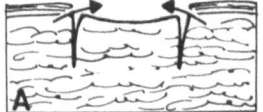 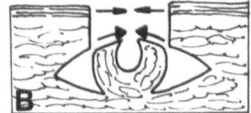 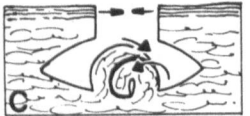

Fig. 29. Carlin and Gurdin's correction of glabellar frown lines. **A** Depressed island is deepithelialized and lateral flaps are overlaid. **B** The central island is deepithelialized and sutured for greater bulk. **C** The central island is deepithelialized and rolled to itself for greater bulk. Fig. 10 from [24], reproduced with permission

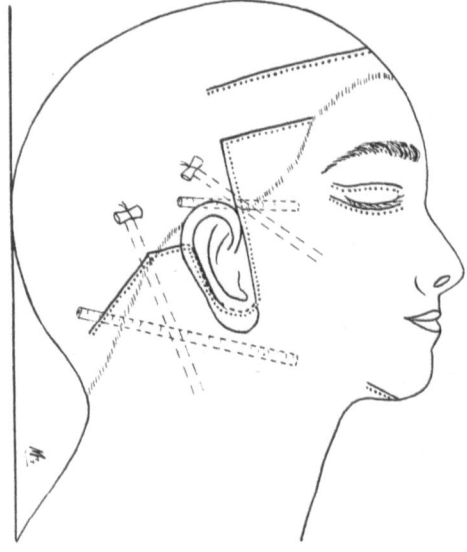

Fig. 30. In 1972 Regnault recommended combining total rhytidectomy, blepharoplasty, rhinoplasty, and mentoplasty within the same operating period. Fig. 4 from [104], reproduced with permission

the tragus in the rhytidectomy for men must not be pulled too close to the ear. To prevent the beard from growing onto the earlobe, a small zone of hairless skin should be left below the incision around the lobe. "By keeping the incisions as short as possible and in the places described," Baker and Gordon observed, "the surgeon will achieve a minor lift, but this seems to be necessary" [3].

Rhytidectomy Developments in the 1970s

In general, recent years have not disclosed any major changes in ways of removing wrinkles and restoring youthfulness [5]. Instead, many of the articles published in the 1970s concerning the removal of wrinkles have emphasized refinements of technique in terms of preliminary tracing, maneuvering tissues, manipulating muscles and musculo-aponeurotic systems, minimizing scars, and dealing with baldness. The necessity for segmental approaches to facial aging has also been reflected in an increasing number of papers, as have the special problems of rhytidectomy in the male and the advisability of combining the

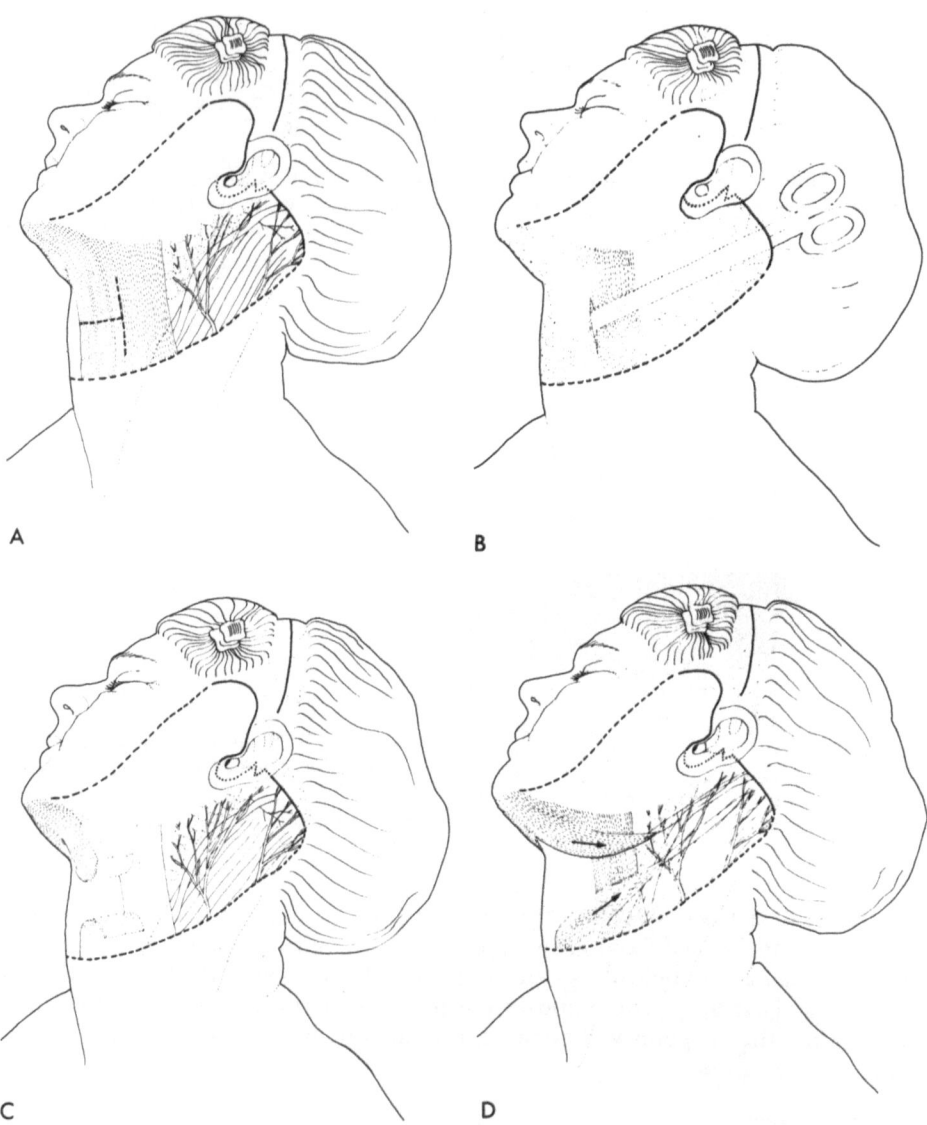

Fig. 31. In 1974 and 1978 Guerrero-Santos published his cervical rhytidectomy, which featured dissection and resuspension of the platysma. **A** Vertical and transverse incision lines in anterior platysma. **B** Detachment of part of platysma. **C** Detached portion of platysma cut transversely to form two flaps. **D** Fastening of flaps to mastoid region with transfixing plication-suspension sutures. From [57], reproduced with permission

rhytidectomy with other procedures within the same operative period. This spate of reports concerned mainly with secondary, combinatory, and refining procedures may be a sign that the major outlines of the rhytidectomy already have been defined. If this is so, then the basic principles deserve at least as

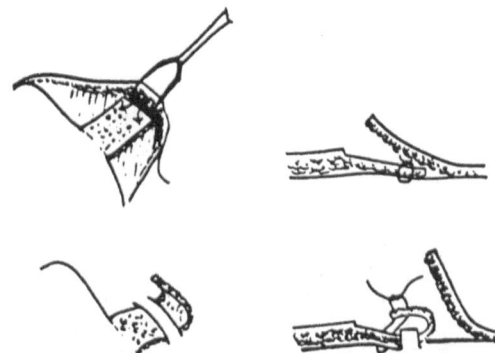

Fig. 32. Cameron et al. developed bucket-handle sutures for secure attachment of dermal flaps in temporal and postauricular areas. Fig. 2 from [22], reproduced with permission

much attention in the future as the refinements of which we read so much.

In 1970 Rodriguez de Lima [105] again recommended a peripheral rhytidectomy performed simultaneously with blepharoplasty. For fine wrinkling around the lip he recommended phenol peeling.

Hinderer [64] wrote in 1970 that he corrects deep wrinkes of the upper lip by means of skin dissection from the muscular layer. The idea is to obviate development of the wrinkles through the temporary implantation of a thin Silastic sheet through an incision at the mucocutaneous juncture on both sides of the columella (Fig. 26). The sheet, surrounded by connective tissue, is removed 1–2 months later.

In 1971 Carlin and Gurdin presented a catalogue of what they call ancillary procedures [24]. To correct "turkey-gobbler" neck, they remove the excess skin and fat through a vertical incision below the chin; they then follow this with multiple A-plasties or W-plasties (Fig. 27). For drooping and excess skin about the eyebrows, they employ Gurdin's method: an incision is made on the brow and then extended to the hairline as the preliminary to a standard rhytidectomy (Fig. 28). Chemical peeling is endorsed as the most promising treatment for removing fine lines about the face.

To correct glabellar frown lines with deep-set vertical and horizontal depressions, Carlin and Gurdin use a local elliptical excision. The epidermis within the ellipse is removed, and the lateral flaps are undermined to cover the ellipse of dermis, which is left attached in its plane. Sometimes the dermis may be doubled over itself and sutured to produce more bulk (Fig. 29). In lateral undermining of the flaps, the corrugator and procerus muscles are partially excised. In further techniques the surgeons include simple undermining of the frown lines by means of a minute incision immediately below the furrows, and perfusion of silicone to enhance the bulk of the glabellar area. In the deeper grooves of the central forehead, a direct elliptical excision is sometimes used to correct the horizontal lines. This is followed by surgical dermabrasion of the skin, and silicone is injected as a filler.

For ptosis of the upper third of the face, Carlin and Gurdin's incision extends inside the hairline in the temporal region and downward along the preauricular region. Undermining and elevation are upward and to the rear.

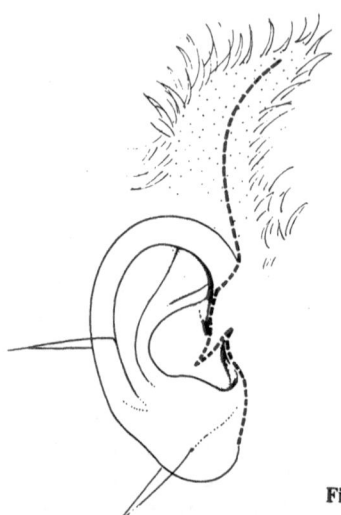

Fig. 33. Stark's preauricular incision is designed to minimize the operative scar. From [117], reproduced with permission

During the 1970s the signs of aging over time were studied and classified by González-Ulloa, Simonin, and Flores [51], and the need for a sectional and/or segmental analysis of the areas of the face in correcting these signs of aging gained ground. Lewis [76] again classified rhytidectomies into the categories of total, sectional (frontal, malar, cervical), and segmental. Snyder [113] advocated combining any needed form of rhytidectomy with nasal and mental profile-plasty to fully restore a youthful appearance, and Regnault [104] recommended a still more ambitious combination of procedures—total rhytidectomy, blepharoplasty, rhinoplasty, and mentoplasty—within the same operating period (Fig. 30).

In the cervical segment, Fredericks [39] advocated concentration of surgical technique in the lower portion of the face, on the ground that aging is less severe, and surgery more hazardous, in the upper frontal segment. For male patients, Fredericks [39] and Carlin and Gurdin [24] endorsed an incision running from the preauricular area toward the canthus of the eye. In the segment of the glabella, Rosenthal [107] has employed an inverted T incision to abolish frown wrinkles and lift the nose; however, the technique draws the two eyebrows together without the improvement of elevating them.

The most important development in rhytidectomy of the cervical segment has concerned the platysma muscle. To sharpen the submandibular-cervical angle more permanently, a recent change has been to dissect this muscle and then to fix it in a more elevated position. Since the platysma is a cutaneous muscle, however, the necessity of this innovation has yet to be confirmed.

The idea of working on the platysma as a separate entity of the skin to improve the results of rhytidectomy was initially explored in reports by Adamson et al. [1], Weisman [126], and Guerrero-Santos and associates [57], and in Skoog's 1974 text [112]. These investigators observed that the skin and adipose in the lower portion of the face and neck constitute a morphologic entity with the superficial fascia and the platysma. With aging, the interconnected skin and platysma shift together, causing sagging of the face and neck. Attention to the platysma and to the superficial musculo-aponeurotic system described by Mitz and Peyronie [91] has caused many speculations and operative innovations [25, 26, 56, 96, 103, 127], adding to rhytidectomy what seems to be promising improvement. In two examples of these new operations published by Connell [25] and Davis [28], excess adipose tissue is resected and a flap of the upper portion of the platysma is sectioned and rotated upward to the internal part of the neck, thus causing the muscular bands to disappear and emphasizing the submandibular-cervical angle. The similar current platysma operation employed by Guerrero-Santos [57] is presented in Figure 31.

In the frontal segment, the value of the coronal incision [51] in obtaining an improved rhytidectomy has been widely recognized in recent years. Gleason's approach [44] to rejuvenation of the frontal segment, for example, is based on a temporal-coronal incision on each side of the head, but he leaves the middle third of the forehead over the nose, unaltered [44]. A procedure designed to remove persistent forehead wrinkles (those that survive manual traction), to correct ptosis or downward slant of the eyebrows, to abolish crow's-feet, and to eliminate frown wrinkles from the glabellar region in a single operation has been described by Viñas, Caviglia, and Cortiñas [124]. After undermining the frontal area, they excise the aponeurotic muscle strips at a level about 3.5 cm above the eyebrow; they resect the corrugator muscle; and, for badly drooping eyebrows, they detach the brow from the orbital rim. All these procedures are performed under local anesthesia. The approach of Le Roux and Jones [74] to rejuvenation of the frontal segment does not involve incision of skin. Instead, they advocate abolishing the frontal muscles.

For the malar region, an operation under local anesthesia has been described by Spadafora, Durand, and de los Rios [115]. A somewhat rounded quadrangle of skin is removed from just in front of the pinna, with undermining carried out as far forward as necessary.

Some interesting refinements of rhytidectomy have been introduced during the 1970s. First, for permanence of traction, Cameron, et al. [22] use mattress sutures to attach dermal flaps in the temporal and postauricular areas to the fascia; they also describe secure attachment of the flaps using a bucket-handle suture (Fig. 32). Second, instead of conforming to the standard face-lift incision in front of the tragus and the helical crus, Stark [117], following the same trend as Meyer [87], has devised a trace that runs along the crest of the tragus and then in front of the helix crus (Fig. 33). Third, neat shaping of the earlobe, accomplished by removing or interpolating a section of skin, has been devised by Loeb [81]. Finally, many innovative operations to correct segmental problems have been described, such as the punch rhinoplasty to elevate the nose [49, 50] or the lipectomy to correct the drooping chin [47].

The value of hormone therapy [48] to halt or decrease the process of aging in the skin has also been a subject of discussion during the 1970s.

In regard to rhytidectomy for the male, Sturman [119] has emphasized an incision that will preserve the non-hair-bearing zone of skin in front of the auricle. He prefers to leave minor signs of scarring rather than to draw the beard-carrying area next to the ear. Hamilton's incision in male rhytidectomy begins at the same place as the usual incision for the female, contouring the lobule, but then it rises into the occipital region and features a prolongation toward the upper lid [62]. Hamilton reported that of 500 rhytidectomies he has performed, 3% were for men; his male patients cited business reasons but Hamilton observed that 2 of the 15 were retired and 4 had younger wives.

Writing on blepharoplasty, Hugo and Stone [68] have pointed out that multiple incisions in the orbicularis oris muscle and the orbital septum for removal of intraorbital fat in blepharoplasty are unnecessary; their anatomic research indicates that the intraorbital fat is not compartmentalized. Tomlinson and Hovey [122] have also written on the matter of adipose in relation to lower lid blepharoplasty. Executed well, their transconjunctival incision for removal of fat from the lower lid seems a clean, ischemic procedure. Berry [7] uses a surgical approach leading directly to the septum when orbital fat has not broken through into the orbicularis muscle. He employs the skin-muscle flap for elevation of the lower lid.

One of the largest classes of articles on the face-lift in the 1970s has been concerned with complications. A statistical study carried out by McGregor disclosed 16.5% major complications in 524 face-lifts, with hematoma accounting for approximately half of them [82].

Baker, Gordon, and Mosienko published a statistical profile of rhytidectomy in 1977 [4]; their analysis covered 1500 rhytidectomies performed between 1959 and 1974. The years 1966 to 1974 showed a stunning increase in cases. The number of male and younger patients also showed an increase, but the percentage in recent years has not changed, and their average age has remained constant—about 56 years. Fifteen percent of patients were repeats, with half of these having had their earlier work performed by the same surgeons; 18.3% of patients coming for rhytidectomy had had earlier aesthetic plastic surgery of some other kind. The major sources of referral were previous satisfied patients. With respect to complications, 15.6% of the cases involved hematoma, 3% being large hematoma and 4.2% hematoma serious enough to warrant return to the operating room for drainage. Baker, Gordon, and Mosienko recommend an office-clinic setting for rhytidectomy, in order to be able to observe the patient for early detection of hematoma [4].

In 1978 Thompson and Ashley [121] reported their series of 922 rhytidectomies performed over a 6-year period. Skin slough necessitating scar revision occurred in 14% of their patients, hematoma in 5%, and seventh nerve injury in 0.7%. Of the 44 patients who developed hematoma, 38 required further aspiration of blood or had unsatisfactory scarring. There was a definite tendency for all complications to occur on the left side (60%), a finding the surgeons initially attributed to their operative sequence; however, changing the sequence to allow for "second-look" inspection of the left side did not change the prevalence of left-sided complications, and Thompson and Ashley now have no explanation for this finding.

A number of surgeons, including Webster [125], report up to 30 ml blood normally lost in a standard malar rhytidectomy. Webster attributes his own success in ischemic operation to elevation of the patient's head, priority use of local anesthesia, and the combined use of meperidine and diazepam. In fact, transoperative management of the patient is a broad problem that requires team assistance and expert knowledge of facial anatomy on the part of the surgeon.

A new form of scissors described by Harley [63] permits easier dissection with less danger of damage to skin, vessels, and nerves. Morgan [92] has recommended omitting bandages following rhytidectomy, because they conceal expanding hematomas.

Complications in blepharoplasty are blindness, ectropion, and damage to the lachrymal tissues—the so-called dry-eye problem. Two papers by Thomas Rees [101, 102] properly recommend meticulous prevention through the most scrupulous management of tissues, avoiding trauma to the ocular conjunctiva. For ectropion, he counsels a 1-month waiting period before applying a full-thickness skin graft if this procedure cannot be performed within 48 hours after blepharoplasty. Obstbaum and Podos [95] reduce intraocular pressure by compression and then prevent its sudden rebounding by means of intraperitoneal administration of indomethacin or simply by peroral aspirin.

Conclusion

Between Cantrell [23] and Cabanès [21] in the first decade of this century and the many practitioners of contemporary rhytidectomy, the concerns and labors of aesthetic plastic surgeons have a familiar tone. We have inherited their improvements and need not waste efforts which theirs have spared us in techniques. Only if we are also the grateful heirs of their subjective scientific and humanistic ideals can we carry forward surgical research to the goals implicit in their pioneering—the safe and effective prolongation of youth and retardation of aging.

The evolution of aesthetic plastic surgery to its present status as a rigorously controlled medical technique received its power from the perennial drive of men and women to preserve the appearance of their body and face in consonance with the vigor of their personalities and desires. We have always known that inner psychic and spiritual changes bring about a new external radiance, but we are now discovering that the process also works in reverse: Change the external appearance—restore the lost years—of a person struggling continually against indifferent or negative social reactions, and the inner light that has died within begins to glow once more.

References

1. Adamson JE, Horton CH, Crawford HH: The surgical correction of the "turkey gobbler" deformity. Plast Reconstr Surg 34:598, 1964
2. Baker TJ: Chemical face peeling and rhytidectomy: A combined approach for facial rejuvenation. Plast Reconstr Surg 29:199, 1962
3. Baker TJ, Gordon TJ: Rhytidectomy in males. Plast. Reconstr Surg 44:219, 1969
4. Baker TJ, Gordon HL, Mosienko P: Rhytidectomy: A statistical analysis. Plast Reconstr Surg 59:24, 1977

5. Baker TJ, Gordon HL, Whitlow DR: Our present technique for rhytidectomy. Plast Reconstr Surg 52:323, 1973
6. Bames OH: Truth and fallacies of face peeling and face lifting. Med J Rec 126:86, 1927
7. Berry EP: Planning and evaluating blepharoplasty. Plast Reconstr Surg 54:257, 1974
8. Bettman AG: Plastic and cosmetic surgery of the face. Northwest Med 19:205, 1920
9. Booth FA: Cosmetic surgery of face, neck, and breast. Northwest Med 21:170, 1922
10. Bourguet J: La disparition chirugicale des rides et plis du visage. Bull Acad Méd 82:183, 1919
11. Bourguet J: Les hernies graisseuses de l'orbite. Notre traitement chirurgical. Bull Acad Méd (3ᵉ Ser.) 92:1270, 1924
12. Bourguet J: Chirugie esthétique de la face: les nez concaves, les rides, et les "poches" sous les yeux. Arch Prov Chir 28:293, 1925
13. Bourguet J: La chirurgie esthétique de la face. Les rides. Monde Méd 38:41, 1928
14. Bourguet J: Notre traitement chirurgical de "poches sous les yeux" sans cicatrice. Arch Franco-Belges Chir 31:133, 1928
15. Brendler R: Beiträge zur korrektiven Dermatologie: II Mitteilung. Die operative Behandlung der Lidfalten. Hautarzt 5:468, 1954
16. Brown AM: Surgical correction of senescent pendulous cheeks. J Int Coll Surg 12:154, 1949
17. Brown AM: Surgical restorative art for the aging face: Notes on the artistic anatomy of aging. J Gerontol 8:173, 1953
18. Brown AM: A prosthetic device for facial rhitidosis. Eye Ear Nose Throat Mon 34:182, 1955
19. Burian F: Zur Technik der Gesichtshautspannung. Med Welt 10:930, 1936
20. Buttkewitz H: Die Nadeltechnik der subkutanen Gewebsraffung, einer schnittlosen Korrekturmethode bei kosmetischen Brust- und Gesichtsoperationen. Zentralbl Chir 81:1185, 1956
21. Cabanès A: Comment naissent et disparaissent: les rides. J Santé May 24, 1903, p 402–404
22. Cameron RR, Litton C, Conrad RN, Latham WD: Use of dermal flaps for attachment of rhytidoplasty flaps. Plast Reconstr Surg 51:596, 1973
23. Cantrell JA: Wrinkles, facial expression a cause—treatment. Am J Dermatol 6:97, 1902
24. Carlin A, Gurdin MM: Ancillary procedures for the aging face and neck. Surg Clin North Am 51:371, 1971
25. Connell BF: Cervical lifts: The value of platysma muscle flaps. Ann Plast Surg 1:34, 1978
26. Connell BF: Contouring the neck in rhytidectomy by lipectomy and a muscle sling. Plast Reconstr Surg 61:376, 1978
27. Cook TE: Rhytidectomy. Dallas Med J 30:60, 1944
28. Davis AD: Obligations in the consideration of meloplasties. J Int Coll Surg 24:567, 1955
29. Davis J: In: Transactions of the Sixth International Congress of Plastic and Reconstructive Surgery, Paris, 1975
30. Edgerton MT, Webb WL Jr, Slaughter R, Meyer E: Surgical results and psychosocial changes following rhytidectomy. An evaluation of face lifting. Plast Reconstr Surg 33:503, 1964
31. Ehrenfeld H: Neue Gesichtspunkte in der Frage der Hängewangenplastik und ein neues Verfahren. Zentralbl Chir 64:202, 1937
32. Eitner E: Indikation und Technik kosmetischer Faltenkorrekturen im Gesicht. Wien Klin Wochenschr 41:1281, 1928
33. Eitner E: Weitere Mitteilungen über kosmetische Faltenoperation im Gesicht. Wien Med Wochenschr 85:244, 1935
34. Erich JB: Rhytidoplasty (face-lift) for wrinkles and redundant tissues about the face and neck. J Staff Meet Mayo Clin 36:68, 1961
35. Farina R: Rugas da face e pescoço (degereraçáo ou atrofia senil da pele do segmento cervico-facial): ritidectomia. Rev Paul Med 64:93, 1964
36. Fischer A: Sul trattamento chirurgico delle rughe del volto: La ridectomia (contributo personale). Policlinico (Chir) 70:335, 1963
37. Fomon S, Bell JW, Schattner A: Aging skin: A surgical challenge. Arch Otolaryngol 61:554, 1955
38. Fomon S, Bell JW, Schattner A, Syracuse V: Aging face: Surgical management. Arch Otolaryngol 73:153, 1961

39. Fredericks S: The lower rhytidectomy. Plast Reconstr Surg 54:537, 1974
40. Frühwald V: Über einen Fall von Hängewange behoben durch eine Modifikation der Joseph'schen Operation. Wien Med Wochenschr 33:1336, 1922
41. Fuchs E: Ueber Blepharochalasis (Erschlaffung der Lidhaut). Wien Klin Wochenschr 91:109, 1896
42. Fuchs E: Textbook of Ophthalmology, 8th ed. Translated by Duane A. Philadelphia, Lippincott, 1924
43. Galand A: Vérités sur la chirugie esthétique et le rajeunissement. Avenir Med 45:8, 1948
44. Gleason MG: Brow lifting through a temporal scalp approach. Plast Reconstr Surg 52:141, 1973
45. González-Ulloa M: Wrinkle correction: Ear-island method. J Int Coll Surg 25:620, 1956
46. González-Ulloa M: Facial wrinkles: Integral elimination. Plast Reconstr Surg 29:658, 1962
47. González-Ulloa M: Ptosis of the chin: The witches' chin. Plast Reconstr Surg 50:54, 1972
48. González-Ulloa M: The ancillary effects of estrogen therapy after rhytidectomy (letter). Plast Reconstr Surg 56:203, 1975
49. González-Ulloa M: Punch rhinoplasty: A complement to rhytidectomy. Aesthet Plast Surg 2:291, 1978
50. González-Ulloa M: Rhinoplastia punch. C P Iberolatinoam 4, April–June, 1978
51. González-Ulloa, Dimonin F, Flores E: The anatomy of the ageing face. In Hueston JT (ed.): Transactions of the Fifth International Congress of Plastic and Reconstructive Surgery (Melbourne, 22–26 February 1971). Sydney: Butterworths Australia, 1971, p 1059–1066
52. González-Ulloa M, Stevens E: Senility of the face—basic study to understand its causes and effects. Plast Reconstr Surg 36:239, 1965
53. González-Ulloa M, Stevens E: Rhytidectomy and related procedures to correct the cau͙es of the appearance of facial senility. Int Surg 49:361, 1968
54. González-Ulloa M, Stevens E: Sectional rhytidectomy, including a description of rhytidectomy in the male. Presented at the 37th meeting of the American Society for Plastic and Reconstructive Surgery, New Orleans, 1968
55. González-Ulloa M, Stevens E, Loewe P, de la Cruz JV, Noble G: Preliminary report on the subcutaneous perfusion of demethyl polisiloxane to increase volume and alter regional contour. Br J Plast Surg 20:424, 1967
56. Guerrero-Santos J, Espaillat L, Morales F: Muscular lift in cervical rhytidoplasty. Plast Reconstr Surg 54:127, 1974
57. Guerrero-Santos J: The role of the platysma muscle in rhytidoplasty. Clin Plast Surg 5:29, 1978
58. Gumpert M: Die operative Faltenentfernung. Med Welt 4:219, 1930
59. Halla F: Kosmetische Faltenkorrekturen. Dtsch Aerztezeitung 87: 1927
60. Halla F: Indikationen und Technik kosmetischer Faltenkorrekturen im Gesicht. Wien Klin Wochenschr 41:1442, 1530, 1928
61. Halla F: Die Beseitigung der Altersfalten im Gesicht (Bemerkungen zu der gleichnamigen Arbeit von Prof. Kromayer in Nr. 22 [60]). Dtsch Med Wochenschr 55:1262, 1929
62. Hamilton JM: Rhytidectomy in the male. Plast Reconstr Surg 53:629, 1974
63. Hartley JH Jr: A new face lift scissors. Br J Plast Surg 27:365, 1974
64. Hinderer U: Tratamiento de las arrugas profundas del labio superior mediante implantacion subcutanea temporal de folio de silicona. Rev Esp Chir Plast 3:151, 1970
65. Holländer E: Plastische (kosmetische) Operation: Kritische Darstellung ihres gegenwärtigen Standes. In G and F Klemperer (eds.), Neue Deutsche Klinik. Berlin: Urban & Schwarzenberg, 1932
66. Hollander MM: Cosmetic surgery of the eyelids and forehead. Eye Ear Nose Throat 37:452, 1958
67. Hollander MM: Rhytidectomy: Anatomical physiological and surgical considerations. Plast Reconstr Surg 20:218, 1957
68. Hugo NE, Stone E: Anatomy for a blepharoplasty. Plast Reconstr Surg 53:381, 1974
69. Johnson JB: The problem of the aging face. Plast Reconstr Surg 15:117, 1955

70. Joseph J: Verbesserung meiner Hängewangenplastik (Melomioplastik). Dtsch Med Wochenschr 54:567, 1928
71. Kromayer F: Die Beiseitigung der Altersfalten im Gesicht: Wundheilung ohne Wundnaht. Dtsch Med Wochenschr 55 [Nr. 22]:912, 1929
72. Krushinski GV, Pakovich GI: Operative elimination of wrinkles of the face and neck. Khirurgiia (Moskva) 38:113, 1962
73. Lagarde M: Cirugía estética de la cara. Cron Med Lima 38:321, 1921
74. Le Roux P, Jones SH: Total permanent removal of wrinkles from the forehead. Br J Plast Surg 27:359, 1974
75. Lewis GK: The surgical treatment of wrinkles. Arch Otolaryngol 60:334, 1954
76. Lewis JR: Segmental approach to rhytidectomy. Plast Reconstr Surg 56:297, 1975
77. Lexer E: Die gesamte Wiederherstellungschirurgie. Leipzig: Barth, 1931
78. Litton C: Chemical face lifting. Plast Reconstr Surg 29:371, 1962
79. Litton C: Observations after chemosurgery of the face. Plast Reconstr Surg 32:554, 1963
80. Litton C, Capinpin A, Portillo A, Pulido F: What we now know about chemosurgery of the face. Presented at the Annual Meeting of the American Society for Aesthetic Plastic Surgery, March 23, 1977, Los Angeles, Calif
81. Loeb R: Earlobe tailoring during facial rhytidoplasties. Plast Reconstr Surg 49:485, 1972
82. McGregor M: Complications of face lifting. In Hueston JT (ed): Transactions of the Fifth International Congress of Plastic and Reconstructive Surgery (Melbourne, 22–26 February 1971). Sydney: Butterworths Australia, 1971, pp 1091–1101
83. Malbec EF: Arrugas de la cara: Téchnica operatoria. Semana Med 111:517, 1957
84. Marino H: Ritidectomia frontal. Bull Soc Cir (Buenos Aires) 47:93, 1963
85. Mayer DM, Swanker WA: Rhytidoplasty. Plast Reconstr Surg 6:255, 1950
86. Mayer DM, Swanker WA: The present status of rhytidoplasty. J Int Coll Surg 25:613, 1956
87. Meyer R: Dauerhaftigkeit, Gefahren and misserfolge kosmetischer Eingriffe im Gesichtsbereich. Aesthet Med 13:273, 1964
88. Millard DR, Pigott RW, Hedo A: Submandibular lipectomy. Plast Reconstr Surg 41:513, 1968
89. Miller CC: The eradication by surgical means of the nasolabial line. Ther Gaz (Detroit) 23:676, 1907
90. Miller CC: Subcutaneous section of the facial muscles to eradicate expression lines. Am J Surg 21:235, 1907
91. Mitz V, Peyronie M: The superficial musculo-aponeurotic system (SMAS) in the parotid and cheek area. Plast Reconstr Surg 58:80, 1976
92. Morgan BL: The aftercare of rhytidectomies with the "no-dressing" technique (letter). Plast Reconstr Surg 51:576, 1973
93. Neuernbergk W: Face-lifting operations. Presented at the 8th Congress of the Deutsche Gesellschaft für die Aesthetische Medizin, 1963. Aesthet Med May, 1963, p 145
94. Noël S: La Chirurgie Esthétique: Son Rôle Sociale. Paris: Masson, 1926
95. Obstbaum SA, Podos SM: Axoplasmic transport (editorial). Invest Ophthalmol 13:81, 1974
96. Owsley JQ Jr: Platysma-fascial rhytidectomy: A preliminary report. Plast Reconstr Surg 60:843, 1977
97. Pangman WJ, Wallace RM: Cosmetic surgery of the face and neck. Plast Reconstr Surg 27:544, 1961
98. Passot R: La chirurgie esthétique des rides du visage. Presse Méd 27:258, 1919
99. Passot R: Quelques généralités sur l'opération correctice des rides du visage (soins prét postopératoire, anesthésie, antisepsie, pensements, soins dermatologiques, irradiation préventive. Rev Chir Plast 3:23, 1933
100. Pires D: Kosmetische Chirurgie der Gesichtsrunzeln. Fortschr Med 52:576, 1934
101. Rees T: Correction of ectropion resulting from blepharoplasty. Plast Reconstr Surg 50:1, 1972
102. Rees T: The dry eye complication after blepharoplasty. Plast Reconstr Surg 56:375, 1975
103. Rees TD, Aston SJ: A clinical evaluation of the results of submusculoaponeurotic dissection and fixation in face lifts. Plast Reconstr Surg 60:851, 1977

104. Regnault P: Complete face and forehead lifting with double traction on "crow's-feet." Plast Reconstr Surg 49:123, 1972
105. Rodriguez de Lima A: Ritidectomia. Rev Lat Am Chir Plast 14(1):37, 1970
106. Rogers BO: A chronologic history of cosmetic surgery. Bull NY Acad Med (sec. ser.) 47:265, 1971 and: The development of aesthetic plastic surgery; A history. Aesth. Plast. Surg., 1:3, 1976
107. Rosenthal SG: Glabellar rhytidoplasty: A new approach. Plast Reconstr Surg 50:36, 1972
108. Schlesinger. Ueber Gesichtsplastiken (Bemerkungen zum Aufsatz von Kromayer in Nr. 22 [60]). Dtsch Med Wochenschr 55:1512, 1929
109. Seltzer AP: Reconstructive surgery for the elderly. Geriatrics 7:185, 1952
110. Serson-Neto D: Rhytidoplasties: Study of 170 consecutive cases. J Int Coll Surg 42:208, 1964
111. Sichel J: Une discussion sur la blépharoplastique. Gaz Hôp 8:276, 1934
112. Skoog T: Plastic Surgery—New Methods and Refinements. Philadelphia: Saunders, 1974
113. Snyder GB: Cervicomentoplasty with rhytidectomy. Plast Reconstr Surg 54:404, 1974
114. Spadafora A: Doble mentón (adiposis submentoniana). Prensa Med Argent 42:1290, 1955
115. Spadafora A, Durand AS, de los Rios E: Flaccidity of the cheeks: Cutaneous resection, with a quadrangular pre-auricular incision. Prensa Univ (Argent) 6:8361, 1975
116. Spira M, Gerow FJ, Hardy SB: Cervicofacial rhytidectomy. Plast Reconstr Surg 40:551, 1967
117. Stark RB: A Variation in rhytidectomy incision at the front of the ear. Plast Reconstr Surg 54:369, 1974
118. Stein RO: Indikation und Technik kosmetischer Faltenkorrekturen im Gesichte. Wien Klin Wochenschr 40:1168, 1927
119. Sturman MJ: Sideburn relationship in the male face lift. Plast Reconstr Surg 57:248, 1976
120. Talamás I: Face lifting (rhytidoplasty). J Am Med Wom Assoc 19:666, 1964
121. Thompson DP, Ashley FL: Face-lift complications: A study of 922 cases performed in a 6-year period. Plast Reconstr Surg 61:40, 1978
122. Tomlinson FB, Hovey LM: Transconjunctival lower lid blepharoplasty for removal of fat. Plast Reconstr Surg 56:314, 1975
123. Uchida JI: A method of frontal rhytidectomy. Plast Reconstr Surg 35:218, 1955
124. Viñas JC, Caviglia C, Cortiñas JL: Forehead rhytidoplasty and brow lifting. Plast Reconstr Surg 57:445, 1976
125. Webster G: The ischemic face-lift. Plast Reconstr Surg 50:560, 1972
126. Weisman PA: Simplified technique in submental lipectomies. Plast Reconstr Surg 48:443, 1971
127. Wood RW: Face lifting with suspensory restoration of the fibromuscular tissues of the face and neck. Aesthet Plast Surg 2:103, 1978

History of Rhinoplasty

Frank McDowell M.D.

Honolulu Hawaii

Until well into the 19th century nasal surgery was confined to the immediate care of acute injuries and to the flap restoration of parts cut off or destroyed by disease.

Perhaps the earliest report of nasal surgery is the description of the treatment of nasal fractures in the *Edwin Smith Surgical Papyrus* (*ca.* 3000 BC) (16) in which the first use of pressure dressings in surgery is found. In India, one of the Brahman holy books, the Sushruta Veda (*ca.* 600 BC) (196) describes the repair of mutilated noses by a cheek flap, using a leaf as a pattern. The work was done by tile-makers and was apparently quite common, due to the practice of cutting off the tip of the nose as punishment (121).

In the writings of the Greek, Roman, Middle-Age, and Renaissance surgeons, nasal surgery was considered only as regards the repair of acute injuries.

Making noses from flaps

The Brancas in Sicily (*ca.* 1430 AD) apparently originated the arm flap reconstruction of noses. This work was carried farther by Gaspare Tagliacozzi and published by him in 1597 (see Gnudi and Webster's (63) excellent monograph on Tagliacozzi).

In 1794 there appeared in the Gentleman's Magazine (123) (in London) a letter from India describing the forehead flap reconstruction of a mutilated nose, together with drawings of the patient (Cowasjee) and the procedure. This letter was signed simply "B.L.," but there is some evidence that the author was a Mr. Lucas (130), an English surgeon who was then resident in Madras, and who later performed the Indian rhinoplasty himself. According to Keegan (84), who later investigated the subject, there is no literature in India between the Sushruta Veda of 900 BC and the 1794 AD letter of "B.L." that would indicate that anything other than cheek flap reconstructions had been done up to the latter time.

A London surgeon, Mr. Joseph C. Carpue (27), took up this work, practiced it successfully, taught it, and wrote a famous small book about it (1816). He also investigated the "B.L." letter about Cowasjee, and obtained the following information.

Lieutenant-Colonel Ward, of the India Service, but at this time resident in London, was the commanding officer of Cowasjee at the time when the latter was mutilated by

From the Division of Plastic Surgery of the University of Hawaii School of Medicine.
Address reprint requests to: Frank McDowell, M.D. Alexander Young Building, Honolulu, Hawaii 96813, USA

0364-216X/78/0001-0321 $05.60
© 1978 Springer-Verlag New York Inc.

the order of Tippoo Sultan and also witnessed the operation performed for restoring the nose. This gentleman has done me the honor to communicate the following particulars.

Cowasjee and four other native soldiers were made prisoners by a marauding party of Tippoo Sultan. The enemy cut off the hands and noses of all the five and then sent them back to the English, with leaves bound over the stumps of their arms to stop the bleeding, but with the remains of their noses as they were left by the knife. In this deplorable state they entered Poonah. The wounds were healed and pensions granted to the unhappy sufferers.

Some time had elapsed, when one day at Poonah a native merchant came to the house of Sir Charles Warre Malet, the British resident at that city, offering for sale oilcloth, and stating his place of residence to be four hundred miles from Poonah. A cicatrix or scar being observed on the centre of the merchant's nose, he was asked how he came by it; upon which he showed another scar on his forehead and explained the operation he had undergone. He confessed that he had been deprived of his nose by the executioner as a punishment for adultery; and added that his new one was the work of an artist who lived where he resided and who frequently did the same for others.

Upon receiving this account, and immediately thinking of Cowasjee and his other fellows, Sir Charles Malet caused the operator to come to Poonah, where he gave new noses to all the five. It was understood at Poonah that this operator was the only one in India; but that the art had been hereditary in his family.

Ambroise Paré, writing in the 16th century, mentioned a patient on whom the Tagliacotian operation was successfully performed and who had for some time previously worn a silver nose. Keegan (84) also told of the Sultan of Turkey supplying silver noses to some of his soldiers whose noses had been cut off by their Bulgarian captors during the war between Russia and Turkey, in 1876. The men were to be seen walking about Istanbul, wearing their silver noses.

Both the arm-flap and forehead-flap reconstructions were taken up by numerous German surgeons in the 19th century, and many variations were developed and tried. During the same time, a number of French surgeons experimented with sliding cheek flaps. The various operations became known as Indian, Italian, or French rhinoplasty.

Johann Friedrich Dieffenbach (43) was probably the greatest master of plastic surgery in the 19th century, and his 1845 edition of *Operative Chirurgie* contains more than 100 pages on flap reconstruction of noses. Contemporary respect for him was so great that all hospitals in Paris were made available to him for operating during his visits there, and all plastic surgeons who have followed him must owe him a great debt. With great lucidity and in considerable detail, he described many varieties of total and partial reconstructions with various flaps.

Dieffenbach recognized the importance of carefully designing the flap, the preparation of the stump to receive the flap, and the postoperative details—as well as the actual transference. Many of his remarks are interesting because of the insight they furnish into the surgery of that era, others because they are just as true today as when he wrote them, and others because they are important original observations.

You cut a nose out of a piece of leather. Before you start the operation, you place the leather pattern on the nose by gluing the edges around the stump. If the shape is satisfactory, you spread the pattern on the forehead in such a way that the part which forms the septum comes to lie close to the hair. You have to shave the hair so that it won't get into the wound. During the operation, the patient leans his head against the breast of the assistant, who holds the sides of the head with his hands. And now you begin.

It is easily understandable that under certain circumstances the operation can't be done. Only very young and healthy people with great courage can endure it. And the surgeon must have great experience.

To replace the nose out of the hairy part of the scalp is not very advisable.

It doesn't have to be mentioned that you can cut the nose out of the skin of the forehead, only where there is one. It could be disintegrated. If this is the case, the flap is taken out of the side, or if this isn't possible, you take it out of the arm.

The forming of a whole nose is sort of a uniform process, because it forms an entire new part according to a given shape. Much more difficult is the partial rhinoplasty, since you have to take into account how the parts that are present will correspond with the new.

When the nostrils are too narrow or are grown together, the operation (for correction) is fairly easy. To keep them open is difficult, however. If you cut out the skin or scars, you cause even more constriction.

Jonathan Mason Warren (203) of Boston observed Dieffenbach's work in Europe, and Warren was one of the first American surgeons to report (in 1837) an Indian rhinoplasty.

The book *La Rhinoplastie,* by Ch. Nelaton and Ombredanne (144) in 1904, depicted a large variety of these operations, using almost every conceivable type of flap.

Keegan (84), who had the opportunity to do a large number of forehead-flap reconstructions in India during the latter part of the 19th century, was one of the first to appreciate the necessity of a lining for the new nose, and to design local skin flaps to be turned down and used for this lining. Keegan's work was largely concerned with replacement of the nasal tip, as that was the part commonly cut off in India (Fig. 1).

Lining the flap nose

Other workers, using either forehead or arm flaps, also turned in the lower end of the flap to form the columella and to line the nostrils. However, Sedillot (180) turned up a flap from the upper lip to form the superior part of the new columella. Volkman turned down a triangular flap from the upper part of the nose to line the mid-dorsum, and he covered it with a forehead flap of nearly the shape presently used. Thiersch (200) turned in flaps from the adjacent cheeks and sutured them together in the midline for lining, then covered the nose with a forehead flap. Helferich (70) turned in a flap from one cheek for lining, and used a flap from the other cheek to cover. Küster (89) put on an arm flap, raw side out, for lining; later he brought down a forehead flap for covering. Berger (11), in 1896, turned down a midline glabellar and lower forehead flap for lining, and then applied an arm flap

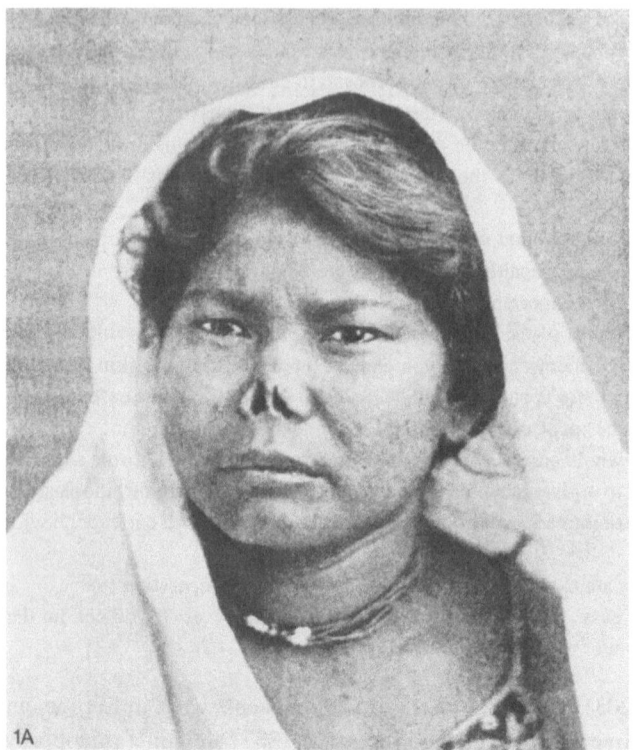

1A

Fig. 1. 19th Century photographs of Indian rhinoplasty. The Hindus usually cut off just the tip of the nose for punishment, and the repair was effected by a flap from the middle of the forehead. (**A**) Preoperative; (**B**) Postoperative (From ref. 84).

for covering. However, Nelaton and Ombredanne (144), who reviewed these various "double flap" operations in 1904, thought that the results of all were bad.

The original Indian or "Koomas" operation was a midline forehead flap twisted down, with no provision for lining.

Collapse of flap noses

With the advent of larger and total nasal reconstructions, the need for a framework became apparent. In 1828, Rousset (144) wrote a thesis in Paris in which he noted the collapse of these noses; he suggested using a framework of gold or silver, to be fixed solidly within the nasal cavity, and that it could be shaped to form a Roman or Carthaginian nose—or even a nose to fit the mode of the day (*à la Roxelanne*).

Nostril collapse and airway tubes

Delpech used metal tubes inside the nostrils to keep the airways open and to support the new nose. Ollier (149) tried using inside removable supports of metal, and also of air balloons. Numerous other removable supports were used in the nasal cavity by various

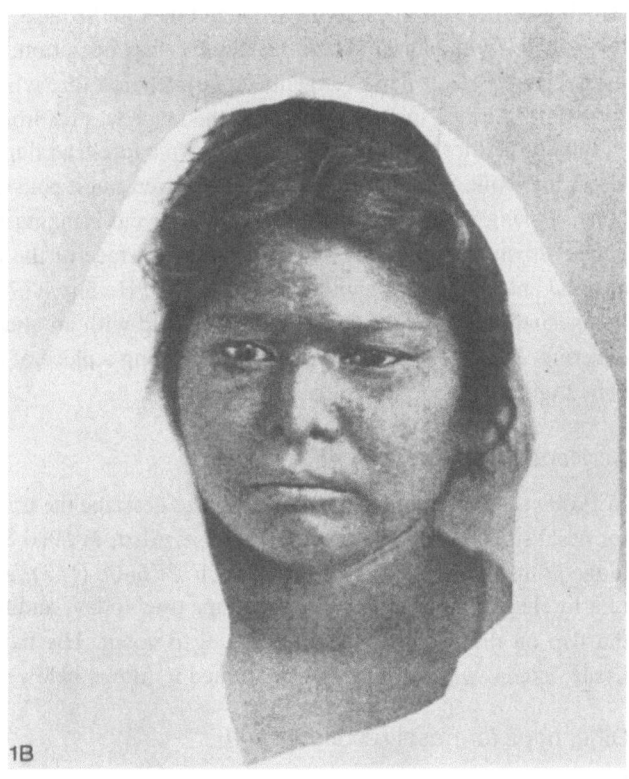

1B

workers. Dieffenbach (43) used gold, Galenzowski lead, Leisrink amber, and Keen one made of silver. Mikulicz used various metals, Lawrence Finny used celluloid, and Lossen and Sauer used caoutchouc (144). These were all removable.

Dorsal collapse and implants for support

Various other workers tried wrapping the flaps around supports which were not removable. In 1877 Despres (144) used such a metallic support. Lotievant used aluminum in 1878. Martin (144), of Lyon, used platinum in the form of a St. Andrew's cross. Most of these supports had some part of the foreign body exposed in the interior of the nose, but in 1887 Delorme (144) devised an operation in which two flaps were used, one for lining and one for covering, with the metal framework in between. Ellison (51) was probably the first to report perforating nasal implants (1894).

Bone grafts for support

Supports made of tissues were also tried. Ollier (149), in 1864, raised periosteum in his forehead flaps to grow new bone in the new nose. Buchanan (25), in England in 1865, reported satisfactory results from this, but Bigelow (13), in Boston in 1867, reported that it was followed by necrosis of the frontal bone. Steinthal (190) used the first jump flap, which was from the chest to the wrist and then to the nose, and he incorporated rib perios-teum in it. Volkman (144), in his double-flap operation, sometimes incorporated peri-osteum in the deep flap. Langenbeck (144) noted that while this transported periosteum sometimes formed microscopic bone; the latter was resorbed later.

In 1864, Ollier (149) tried bringing down a forehead flap with not only periosteum, but also some bone in it. König (87) boldly sawed out a considerable segment of the frontal bone, leaving it attached to the forehead flap and bringing it down with the flap; this was hinged down with the skin on the posterior surface of the new bony septum, which was covered anteriorly with another forehead flap. Helferich (70) turned over a cheek flap for lining, and then brought down a forehead flap with an attached piece of frontal bone for covering. Israel (73) used a wrist flap containing a piece of the ulna, and he also used free bone transplants from the tibia.

Cartilage grafts for support

In 1900 von Mangoldt (116) was the first to describe the transplantation of costal cartilage for nasal support, using it in a saddle nose. Also, in 1900 Steinthal (190) used costal car-tilage in his jump flap from the chest. Ch. Nelaton (143), again in 1900, reported the use of a forehead flap of practically the shape used today, and he transplanted cartilage under the flap on the forehead before bringing it down. His flap was lined only with fibrous tissue, except where the ends were turned in (down below).

Other flaps for nasal reconstruction

In 1920 Gillies (59) reported the use of tubed flaps from the neck and chest, swung on a mastoid pedicle. These were based on his experiences during World War I.

Later, there were a large number of reports showing excellent results from various flaps, and it is difficult to select any particular ones for comment. Sheehan (187) reported the use of a cross-scalp forehead flap for small repairs in 1925. New (145), in 1945, also originated a cross-scalp flap; it was based on a temporal pedicle and transferred to the opposite side of the forehead with minimal residual scarring; he called it the "sickle flap." Other interesting designs included the "up and down" forehead flap, reported by Gillies (61), and the "scalping flap," described by Converse (35).

One of the reports that received considerable attention was by Blair (14), in 1925, on *Total and Subtotal Restoration of the Nose*. Fundamental points he included were: (a) forehead flaps made the best major repairs; (b) the best design is one similar to that of Nelaton, using the entire depth of the forehead and swinging it on a supraorbital pedicle; (c) lining is provided by turning down—or in—any local skin remnants for the upper part—and turning under the lower end of the flap for lining the lower part; (d) cartilage is the best supporting framework; (e) provision and preparation of a good platform for the new nose is an important part of the work.

The beautiful results obtained in many patients in World War II, and since then, illus-trate the culmination of this 2000-year-old story.

Treatment of saddle deformities by skeletal implants and transplants

The early attempts at correction often used skin flaps inserted into the dorsum.

Dieffenbach devised three different operations for local cutting and shifting of tissues on the dorsum, in the 1820–1840 period. But in 1845, in his *Operative Chirurgie* (43), he advised cutting across the nose, pulling it down, and inserting a forehead flap in the upper dorsum. This flap was inserted at first under the nasal skin, with the raw side anterior.

Many other workers devised operations in which pieces of frontal bone were brought down in a forehead flap, as outlined earlier in this paper. Szymanowski (144), Roberts (161), and others cut across the dorsum, pulled the tip down, and inserted cheek flaps in the dorsum.

Other early attempts included the insertion of either removable or nonremovable frameworks of various metals within the nasal cavity to hold the dorsum forward. Apparently, these were used mostly in luetic noses, where the entire septum and bones were missing and there was just one large cavity covered by skin. Such apparatuses were described by Dieffenbach, Mikulicz, Leisrink, Chaput, Monks, Pearse, and others (144). Gold, silver, and platinum were favored metals. Other varieties of apparatus are listed earlier (under methods of supporting flap noses).

Injections of "vaseline" (this may or may not have been similar to present day petrolatum) were described by Gersuny (58); this work was quickly picked up by many others but later discarded because of unfavorable results. Among the complications were severe local reactions and distant emboli, including fatal pulmonary emboli.

The injection of low-melting point paraffins was started in 1904 by Eckstein (144), and this method was used by many workers for 20 years or more. The immediate results appeared good, so numerous syringes were developed and many different materials were tried. The work was finally discarded because of serious paraffinoma formation locally, and because of distant complications (including phlebitis, thrombosis, pulmonary emboli, and infarction).

Subcutaneous transplants or implants into saddle noses were a natural carry-over from their use in flap noses, and these were used by many workers, beginning in the early 19th century. Many different inorganic materials were used, in many shapes, with and without perforations, and later discarded.

The first biologic transplants were the bringing down of periosteum, and later bone, from the frontal area in forehead flaps, as noted before. In 1875, James Hardie (68) first described the insertion of a denuded fifth finger into a saddle nose, later cutting it off and leaving it in the nose. This work was tried and reported by a number of workers, including J.M.T. Finney (53), but was discarded later for obvious reasons.

Heterogenous transplants were tried by many surgeons; one of the most interesting descriptions (Fig. 2) is by Robert Weir (205) in 1892. He described making an inverted-V

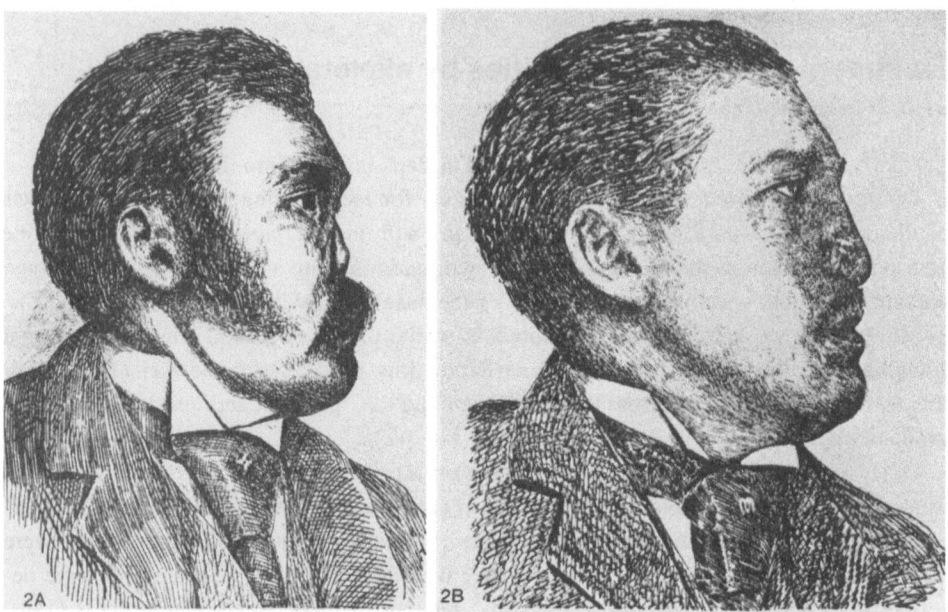

Fig. 2. Interesting case in which a duck's sternum was transplanted into a saddle nose, with later extrusion. (**A**) Preoperative; (**B**) Postoperative. (From ref. 205).

incision on the dorsum of a saddle nose under local anesthesia, and then preparing the subcutaneous bed.

> At this period of the operation a young duck, which had been chosen, was killed, and its breast bone was cut into shape . . . and inserted. The restoration of the nose was remarkably satisfactory. Three weeks passed. The patient's delight was great, and mine was greater. Unluckily, soon after he complained of an increased discharge from his nose. At the end of the seventh week a swelling appeared at the root of the nose culminating in an abscess . . . In brief, at the end of eight weeks I felt that my procedure was not a success, and thought it was necessary to remove this foreign body.

Although written in the 19th century, this seems to be one of the most lucid descriptions of the usual fate of heterogenous and nonbiologic transplants.

The autogenous cartilage transplants from the ribs to the nose, first described by von Mangoldt (116) in 1900, formed the basis for most of the lasting work in this direction. He inserted the cartilage through a glabellar incision.

Autogenous bone transplants from the tibia to the saddle nose were first described by Israel (73) in 1896. This work was later adopted by Joseph (79) and by many others. Israel used a longitudinal incision along the dorsum, but Joseph put the transplant in through an intranasal incision.

Czerny (37), in 1895, reported cutting through each upper lateral cartilage a few millimeters lateral to the septum, then turning the medial ends upward and suturing them back-to-back to elevate the dorsum of a nose. This work was used and reported on later by many authors using several variations [e.g. Maliniac (111), in 1932].

Heterogenous transplants have been reported by many workers using them in different areas, including the nose, for a long time. P.S. Stout (191) reported the use of bovine cartilage in the nose in 1933; this was reported subsequently by González-Ulloa (65) in 1942, and by Gillies and Kristensen (62) in 1951.

Others [including Brown (18) in 1940] tried it, but they encountered violent extrusions.

As noted before, Rousset (144) described in 1828 the introduction of gold and silver skeletons into noses. Following this, there were many descriptions of transplants of these metals or of platinum, aluminum, amber, rubber, ivory, etc. E. F. Malbec of Argentina reported on the use of ivory (97) transplants in 1938, marble (98) transplants in 1940, duraluminum (100) transplants in 1941, bone (99) transplants in 1941, bone (101) transplants in 1942, osteocartilaginous (102) homogeneous grafts in 1943, tantalum (103) in 1946, and the use of preserved cartilage (194) in 1947. From a perusal of the literature and a discussion with other workers, it would seem that this same process has been gone through by many surgeons, though without such complete reporting.

For many years there was considerable controversy over the relative merits of ivory, bone, and cartilage. Vaillancourt (202) (of Canada) used cartilage in 1913. Carter (28) (of New York) used bone in 1914; Rotkitski (164) (of Russia) used bone in 1914; Morestin (140) (of France) used cartilage in 1914; Arkin (3) (of Boston) used bone in 1915; Schilling (176) (of Sweden) used bone in 1915; Levy (91) (of Germany) used bone in 1910. Boyd and Gallie (15) (of Canada) used bone in 1918. Maliniac (105–112) used ivory in 1924 to 1933, and he reported on a comparative study of ivory and organic transplants (105), favoring the use of ivory. Carter (29) again reported on the use of bone and cartilage in 1923. L. Cohen (32) used mixed bone and cartilage grafts in 1927. Dahmann (38) reported the use of cork implants (in Germany) in 1931. Salinger (171) described in 1931 the use of ivory implants in 50 cases. McIndoe (134) used cartilage in 1934; Prudente (156) used ivory in 1934; Safian (168) used ivory in 1935, and Salinger (172) again reported on the use of ivory and on cartilage transplants in 1937. Spanier (188) reported on the use of alloplastic (especially ivory) and heteroplastic grafts in 1936. Alves (2) reported on the use of ivory and of costal grafts in 1936, and M. M. Wolfe (207) used ivory in 1938. Mowlem (141) preferred iliac bone grafts, Young (208) reported on costal cartilage transplants in 1938, and Zeno (210) reported on the use of marble in 1939.

Although there is a dearth of written reports, it is well known that a number of surgeons put in large numbers of bakelite and other plastic implants at about this time, and many plastic surgeons later saw the unfortunate results of these extrusions.

O'Connor and Pierce (148) reported, in 1938, on their use of homogenous rib cartilage, preserved under refrigeration in a merthiolate-saline solution.

J. B. Brown (18) reported, in 1940, on the use of preserved cartilage, and noted that he had used it since 1928 in noses. L. Cohen (33) reported again, in 1940, on the use of mixed bone and cartilage grafts, and Mowlem (142) reported again in 1941 on the use of iliac bone and cartilage in noses. In 1941 New and Erich (147) advocated boiling fresh autogenous cartilage before inserting it into noses to prevent subsequent warping. Straith and Slaughter (195) reported, in 1941, on the use of preserved cartilage. In the same year, Kimball and Drummond (85) described the use of vitallium transplants. S. W. MacCollum (95) reported on the use of iliac bone in 1942. Barksy (9) reported using a molded bone graft in 1945. Peer (152) reported cartilage grafting in 1944 and the following year described experimental observations on the growth of human cartilage (153) and its use in noses. Linhares (93) used vitallium in 1946 and in 1947 Daley (39) reported on the use of boiled cartilage. In 1948 the use of acrylic was described by Holt and Lloyd (72) and by Grasch (66). L. Dufourmentel and Ginested (48) reported two cases the same year and noted that both implants came out. Rapin (157) described 8 years' experience with the use of acrylic in 1949.

J. B. Brown and DeMere (21) described, in 1948, the details of operating a preserved cartilage bank. B. C. Martin (117) reported, in 1948, on the use of cancellous bone grafts and in 1949 Brunner (24) wrote on the fate of autogenous rib cartilage in the nose. Seeley (181) described, in 1948, the use of a composite bone graft in saddle-nose deformities, and Dingman (44), in 1950, reported his experiences with iliac bone grafts in the face. Dupertuis (50) reported, in 1950, on the growth of young human autogenous cartilage grafts in the nose. Vadala and Somers (201) reported, in 1950, on the use of preserved homografts of bone in the nose. Gerrie, Cloutier, and Woolhouse (57) described, in 1950, the use of carved cancellous bone. Wible, Trombetta, and Wineinger (206) described, in 1951, the use of a tantalum mesh in the nose.

In 1948 Rubin, Robertson, and Shapiro (167) reported on the use of polyethylene transplants, and in 1951 Rubin (166) described his experiences with this material over a period of 3 years.

In 1943 Peer (151) reported on the use of diced cartilage grafts, and in 1948 Penn, Jankowitz and Bruewer (155) described their experiences with grated cadaver cartilage; MacMillan (96) introduced a knife with multiple blades for dicing cartilage and DeKleine (41) introduced a "chondrojet" for injecting finely grated cartilage. In 1950 New and Austin (146) reported on a "chondrotome-ejector" for both shredding and injecting cartilage.

The shape of the transplants has varied almost as much as the material. Almost all of the early writers, (including Joseph) used simple dorsal bars put in as cantilevers, and these were usually bone. Cartilage does not unite with bone and may actually depress, rather than support, the nose when it is put in this way. For that reason, various workers tried using columellar struts, but the two-piece transplants often slipped and were unstable. In 1940 J. B. Brown (18) reported on his use of a one-piece "L" shaped cartilage transplant to support and build out the nose. Since then variations of this have been used by many surgeons, though some still prefer bone cantilevers.

Most of the early transplants were put in through glabellar or dorsal incisions. Joseph (79) reported the introduction of bone through an intranasal incision in 1907, and this access is still preferred by some surgeons. Others prefer the columellar splitting incision—particularly if a triangle of "L" shaped cartilage transplant is to be inserted.

Restoration of defects of the alae and tip

In 1845 Dieffenbach (43) suggested turning down a local flap from above the defect for covering, and then bringing down a vertical flap from the middle of the forehead for covering. A little later Labat (144) reported a similar method, using a midline forehead flap but cutting a hole through the nose and sliding down the border of the defect for the new nostril rim. In 1870 Szymanowski (197) described the use of a transverse forehead flap.

Labat (144) [in 1833] and Dieffenbach (43) [in 1845] also described alar repairs with arm flaps.

During the middle and last part of the 19th century, numerous French and German surgeons evolved various plans of repair by shifting local flaps from elsewhere on the nose, the cheeks or the upper lip. These possibilities were pretty well exhausted by Sedillot, Roux, von Langenbeck, Verhaeghe, Verneuil, Duvernoy, Denonvilliers, Alquie, Labat, Mutter, Szymanowski, Dieffenbach, A. Nelaton, Ch. Nelaton, Fritz, Reich, Bonnet, Weber, Blandin, Thompson, Preidlsberger, Bouisson, von Hacker, and others (144). The very multiplicity of the plans, and the lack of popularity of any of them, suggests that none of them were very satisfactory.

Dieffenbach (43) and others also described V-Y and Z-plasty local shifts to decrease the size of the nostril and make a new alar border.

Von Hacker (144) used a three-way combination of a local nose flap, a cheek flap, and a Thiersch skin graft to provide both lining and covering. Ch. Nelaton (144) turned down the edge of the defect for lining, and brought up either a nasolabial flap or an arm flap for cover.

Composite grafts

In 1902 König (88) described a free transplant of both the skin surfaces and the intervening cartilage from the rim of the ear to repair alar defects. This report was lost sight of—possibly because it was just a single suggestion in one paper among many on numerous other impossible or unsatisfactory procedures, or perhaps because it seemed contrary to the then known principles of free grafting. König's suggestion was later reprinted (without documentary results) in at least two books, but not believed. There were no further reports of its actual use during the next 40 years, and throughout this period these repairs were routinely done with the various flaps mentioned above.

In 1943 Gillies (61), apparently just as unaware of König's report as everyone else, described implanting a single-thickness of skin with cartilage from the ear under a forehead flap, and then later bringing the flap with this down to repair an alar defect.

In March of 1946 J. B. Brown and B. C. Cannon (20) reported their use of composite free grafts of cartilage and both thicknesses of skin from the ear to the nose, as used by them during World War II at the Valley Forge General Hospital. Photographs of a number of excellent results were shown, not only in repairs of the ala but also in the columella and about the tip. They, as well as many other surgeons who began using this plan, thought this work to be new—but later König's original report was found. In September of 1946 Dupertuis (49) described a free graft of fat and skin from the lobe of the ear for repair of alar defects.

The great usefulness of the composite graft for these repairs is shown by the widespread use of it in recent years.

The reduction rhinoplasty

In Dieffenbach's *Operative Chirurgie* (43) [1845] there is a brief mention of straightening the twisted nose. The work was done through external incisions, chiseling the bones loose from the face and the septum loose from the palate, then fracturing the nose over into a position of overcorrection.

In 1887 John Roe (of Rochester, N.Y.) presented a paper before the state medical society of New York entitled *The Deformity Termed Pug Nose, and Its Correction by a Simple Operation* (162). In this paper he described the reduction of bulbous nasal tips in 5 patients, and he illustrated the results with before and after sketches (Fig. 3). He did the work through intranasal incisions—dissecting the lining loose, lifting the tip of the nose up, and cutting out the excess bulk. When the alar cartilages were deformed, he trimmed or cross-hatched them. After the operation, he put silver tubes in the nostrils and "molded a saddle or splint" over the outside to hold the nose in its new shape until healing had occurred.

In 1891 Roe presented another paper before the same society, entitled *The Correction of Angular Deformities of the Nose By a Sub-Cutaneous Operation* (163). This was the

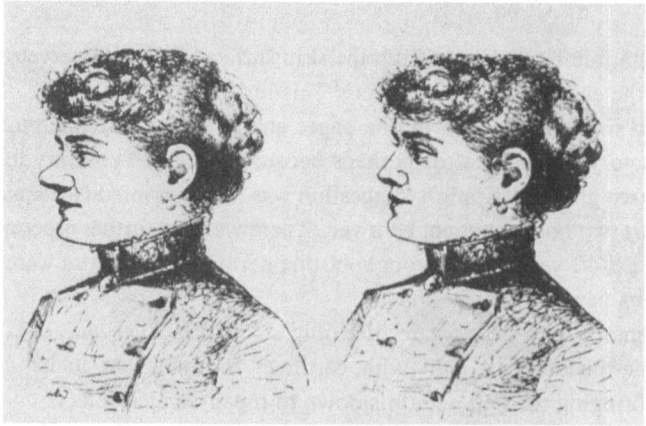

Fig. 3. This illustration of a tip reduction is from the first definitive report of a reduction rhinoplasty. (From ref. 162).

first clear-cut description of nasal hump removal, and it was illustrated by *photographs* of such patients before and after operation (Fig. 4). The work was done under local cocaine anesthesia. He stated, "I made a lineal incision completely through the upper wall of the nostril, just in front of the nasal bone, between it and the upper lateral cartilage of the nostril, to the under side of the skin." It seems possible from some of his other remarks that he was mistaken in his interpretation of the anatomic landmarks, and that he may have made the opening incisions between the upper and lower laterals, as they are often done today. After the initial incisions, he undermined the skin widely and inserted angular bone scissors up through the nostrils to cut the hump off until the dorsum was smooth. Then he strapped the skin down on the new dorsum using a splint under pressure.

The above two papers establish Roe, beyond doubt, as the originator of corrective rhinoplasty.

In 1892 Robert F. Weir of New York City published a paper entitled *On Restoring Sunken Noses* (205). He noted that he had done previous work on these noses with flaps, but here he described a new operation through intranasal incisions in which he chiseled the bones loose from the face, moved them in, and held them with steel needles put transversely through the nose, using shot clamped on the needles on either side.

As a sort of addendum to the above paper, Weir describes a patient, whom he first saw in 1885, with a very large nose—"it seemed to his physicians and relatives essential to the preservation of the balance of his mind to relieve him."

> Weir resected a wedge of the nasal dorsum to lower it, and used a forceps to crush the lower ends of the nasal bones inward. Soon he found that he had become involved in a real problem; the patient was far from satisfied.
>
> At the second operation (2 months later), he did the excision of the nostril bases, which has since been known by his name. Following this, he states that the patient had a "monomania," and was still not satisfied.
>
> At the third operation, he cut across the bases of the alae and the columella, lifted

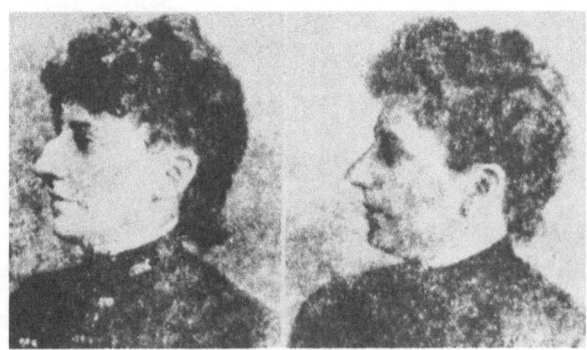

Fig. 4. The first photographic record of an osteoplastic reduction of the nose. (From ref. 163).

the entire nose up, and trimmed the upper lateral cartilages. Still the patient was most unhappy.

The fourth operation consisted of a further hump removal, using a chisel through external skin incisions.

Weir also described two other patients in whom he removed humps through intranasal incisions, and he noted that internal packing or plugs would not permanently change the shape of an operated nose, or hold it up. He concluded with a description of the correction of a flared nostril in a cleft lip patient; for this, he undermined the nostril base, moved it medially, and held it there with a through-and-through stitch, which traversed the columella and the normal alar base.

Weir deserves much credit for the above early, lasting, important contributions to nasal surgery—including the recognition of the unhappy patient who seeks one rhinoplasty after another forevermore.

Monks (139) of Boston, in 1898, described corrective rhinoplasties in which he cut the alar bases and the columella loose from the lip to elevate the nose for better direct vision in trimming. For some reason, this reversion to external incisions was followed by many; unfortunately it retarded the general acceptance of rhinoplastic surgery a great deal. (In 1923 Gillies (60) described an incision in which he cut the columella loose from the lip, then from the septum, and turned it upward for exposure.)

Enter Jacques Joseph

In 1898 an orthopedic surgeon of Berlin, Jacques Joseph, published a paper entitled *Surgical Correction of the Nose* (74), illustrated by sketches of remarkably good results for the time (Fig. 5). When operating, he thought he was the first to do this work, but before publication of his paper he came across the works of Dieffenbach, Weir, and Roe. In this early period, Joseph excised a V-shaped segment along the dorsum—clear through the

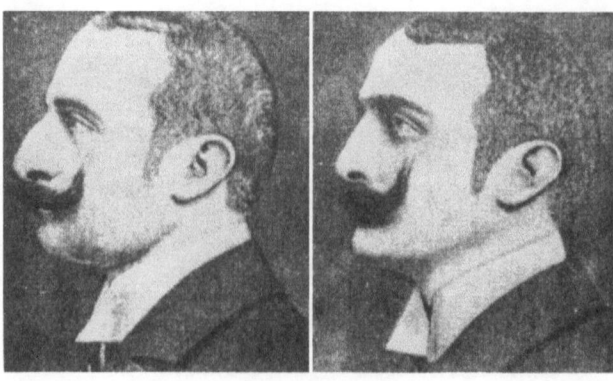

Fig. 5. Illustration of result of rhinoplasty from Joseph's paper on the subject. (From ref. 74).

skin, bone, cartilage and lining—and also took a wedge off the bottom of the septum to shorten the nose.

In 1902 Joseph published a second paper, one entitled *About Some More Operative Nasal Reductions* (75), and he noted that he had now done 10 such operations. He was still doing his rhinoplasties through external skin incisions (removing the hump, and then shortening the nose). He illustrated the plane for removal of the dorsal hump, and he noted that Dr. Rudolf Virchow had examined some of his patients with interest.

In 1904 Joseph published the paper *Intranasal Hump Removal* (76), noting that he now did rhinoplasties through intranasal incisions and had completed 43 cases. In 1904 his article on *Nasal Reductions* (77) was the first to illustrate his intranasal right-angled saws, and also his external clamp (or splint). In 1905 he published *Some More About Nasal Reductions* (78), and noted that he had now operated on 100 such patients. In 1907 he published *The Correction of Twisted Noses* (80) and illustrated his golf-stick knife, together with a number of other intranasal instruments he had designed. In this paper he described mobilization of the displaced septum and wiring it over in place, as well as the use of various headband appliances to help hold it there. At this time he insisted on careful photographic and plaster-cast records for the study of each patient, and to document the results of each operation.

In 1907 Joseph also published his *Treatise on Rhinoplasty* (79), which was an extensive article dealing with many types of nasal deformity, their classification, and the individual operative steps for their correction. In addition to reduction of the nose, he used free bone transplants from the tibia to build up saddle deformities.

These single papers were eventually followed by a lengthy and well illustrated treatise (81) on rhinoplasty in Katz's *Handbuch der Speciellen Chirurgie* [1922], and finally by his monumental monograph *Nasenplastik und sonstige Gesichtsplastic* (82) [1931].

Joseph's position is unique in this work. With only the beginning, halting efforts of Roe and Weir preceding him, he not only pioneered but developed practically the whole field of rhinoplastic surgery. He studied, analyzed, and classified the various types of deformities, devised operative procedures for the correction of each one, and invented instruments with which to do the work. His operative skill and excellent recording then firmly established the various operations. One could almost say that this category of surgery was "born full grown" with the appearance of his book, though there have naturally been many imporant contributions since that time.

Other contemporary writers

During the first quarter of the 20th century, there were many other individual reports of rhinoplastic procedures and results. Some were repetitive, while others introduced procedures which were afterwards abandoned. Many new instruments were described, most of which were either overlooked or discarded. One of the more interesting ones was the tiny motor-driven circular saw devised by Moulonguet (47) [1922] for rhinoplastic work.

Sheehan's first edition of *Plastic Surgery of the Nose* (187) [1925] describes his work done through a columellar-splitting incision, using chisels instead of saws. In his second edition, [1936] he had changed to intranasal incisions, but he still used chisels (a practice continued by his trainees).

In 1932 Maliniac (111) wrote about turning up flaps of upper lateral cartilages to elevate a depressed nasal dorsum, essentially the procedure described by Czerny (37) in 1895.

In 1933 Clare Straith (193) described a "rhinometer" for use in planning cosmetic rhinoplasties.

Later writers on cosmetic rhinoplasty

Joseph Safian deserves great credit for bringing the attention of English-speaking surgeons to the work of Jacques Joseph, and also for a number of additions of his own. His book *Corrective Rhinoplastic Surgery* (168) [1935] is a model of clear writing and description; it resulted in the widespread adoption of Joseph's procedures and the development of acceptable rhinoplastic surgery in this country.

During the second quarter of this century, the number of individual papers on rhinoplasty became voluminous, with many individual variations, suggestions, and improvements. It is almost impossible to determine proper priority for each of these.

In 1940 Maliniac (113) described the prevention and treatment of some late sequelae in rhinoplasty. In 1940 Aufricht (6) noted that whereas Joseph used only adhesive and gauze dressings for rhinoplasties, occasional hematomas followed this; Aufricht carefully described his own method of pressure dressings, using a splint molded out of dental compound.

In 1940 also, J. B. Brown (19) wrote a chapter in Nelson's Loose-Leaf Surgery entitled *Reconstructive Surgery of the Nose*, in which he described his techniques for corrective rhinoplasty, cartilage transplants, the treatment of fractures, flap restorations, cleft lip nasal repairs, and other nasal operations. He used malleable aluminum nasal splints for dressings. In the same year (1940), Converse (34) described some of the currently used procedures on tip cartilages and Cinelli (31) advocated operations on the muscles about the tip for the correction of collapse of the nares (1941). Safian (169) called attention to many common errors in rhinoplasty, their prevention, and their correction by secondary procedures. Straatsma (192) described the removal of a nasal hump and transplantation of it into a forehead defect. Cinelli (30) wrote about some perforated guides for nasal saws and other special instruments he had devised.

In 1941 Scher (175) and others described the transplantation of nasal humps into retruded chins. Metzenbaum (135) and Salinger (173) advocated the use of individually made copper splints after rhinoplasty.

In 1942 W. B. Davis (40) wrote about the correction of various nasal deformities. Parsons (150) and others again advocated the use of plaster-of-paris casts for splinting nasal fractures and after rhinoplasties.

In 1943 Greeley (67) described the treatment of various nasal deformities, abrasions, accidental tattoos, scars, keloids, *etc*. In the same year Berson described a rhinometer not too different from the earlier one designed by Straith (193). An important paper by Aufricht (7), modestly labeled *A Few Hints and Surgical Details in Rhinoplasty*, contained a number of excellent refinements in cosmetic rhinoplasty. These were promptly adopted by many surgeons doing this work. Seltzer (182) also described one of these refinements, out-fracturing of the nasal bones.

In 1944 Salinger (174) reviewed the treatment of traumatic deformities and Lamont (90) discussed various procedures for the correction of congenital and other deformities. Seltzer (183) described hinging out straight various angulations of the septum (a procedure described first by Joseph and later by Metzenbaum).

In 1945 Maliniac (114) again described the procedure for elevating the nasal dorsum by folding up flaps from the upper lateral cartilages.

Straith (194) described elongation of the columella in 1946. In 1947 Herbert (69) described another nasal splint, Steffensen (189) the reconstruction of the nasal septum, and Gatewood (56) expressed his preference for the use of chisels instead of saws.

In 1948 Becker (10) described a special nasal speculum, and Seeley (181) outlined the reconstruction of the nasal tip. Rubin (165) introduced a new intrument, and Rethi (159) wrote an article entitled *Right and Wrong in Rhinoplastic Operations*. Kazanjian (83) discussed the repair of syphilitic deformities, and also noted that he liked to use a nasal hump-cutting scissors rather than saws.

In 1949 Young (209) reviewed the surgical repair of nasal deformities. Pelliciari (154) wrote on columella and tip reconstruction, and Aldunate (1) described a new osteotome.

In 1950 Roberts (160) outlined the treatment of nasal fractures, and Converse (36) reviewed the treatment of deviated noses. Webster and Deming (204) described the surgical treatment of the bifid nose. Berndorfer (12) discussed consideration of the physiognomy in esthetic rhinoplasty, and A. M. Brown (17) discussed the reduction of "elephantiasis nostras nasalis." Ashley and King (4) introduced a new nasal splint. A number of writers, including Fomon (54) and Fred (55), advocated implanting the lower end of the septum between the medial crura of the alar cartilages to prevent secondary drooping of the nasal tip; however, other surgeons felt that this procedure is not normal anatomically, that it produces a much too wide columella, and that the prevention of such secondary drooping should consist of cutting down the dorsal line to the height of the tip.

In 1951 Tamerin (199) reported a case of reconstruction of a nasal fistula, and Cardoso (26) discussed reconstruction after nasal leishmaniasis. May (118) noted that he still preferred the Rethi incision (cutting across the columella) for exposure in cutting down very large noses. Koechlin (86) described new instruments. Bames (8) described his work in elective rhinoplasty, noting that he removed the hump with an osteotome, clipped V-segments out of the tip cartilages, and usually completed the operation in about 20 minutes in his office.

In 1952 Douglas (46) described an operation for relief of vestibular nasal obstruction by partial resection of the nasal process of the maxilla.

In 1952 the first edition of Brown and McDowell's book, *Plastic Surgery of the Nose*, (22), appeared. It covered in detail the anatomy of the nose and the more or less standard rhinoplastic procedures which had been developed during the preceding 60 years on this anatomic basis—ones which had been proven to be good by many plastic surgeons. The book enjoyed a popularity quite unanticipated by the authors and received a large and wide distribution; it has been said that most of the rhinoplasties being done today are being done by men, or their students, who once studied this text.

A sordid chapter

During the late 1940s and early 1950s there was a spate of "quickie" courses on rhinoplasty given by teachers whose abilities were questioned by many, probably most, plastic surgeons of the time. The courses were usually given to nonplastic surgeons, persons who for the most part had never even considered doing any esthetic operation before—but whose practices based on sinus and mastoid infections had fallen apart with the advent of antibiotics. For many, the collapse in their practices occurred while they were away in the military forces in World War II. The Veterans Administration paid their expenses for some of these "quickie" courses, and they seized this paid-for opportunity to move forthwith into another field. Usually these courses lasted for 3 days to 3 weeks—though a few were longer. Frequently, these middle-aged "students" were required to buy a set of rhinoplastic instruments from the instructor (or from a firm which "took care" of the instructor). Some of the teachers would agree to give "the course" any place where, and anytime when, a few paying students and a couple of willing patients could be brought together for a few days.

In some of these courses, there was a good deal of nonsense trumpeted about the air in the left nostril going to the left lung, the air in the right nostril going to the right lung, the air in the left inferior meatus going to the left lower lobe, *etc., etc.* Some of these "teachers" were advocating looking at the patient's chest film, rather than at her nose, while deciding what to do in a rhinoplasty. There was talk about "morcellizing" the cartilages into a "bag of beans," and of cutting the bony part of the nose down to harmonize with the lower half. Much of the real rhinoplastic knowledge that had been painfully and carefully obtained and substantiated duing the preceding 60 years was ignored, not understood, or cast aside—particularly by those persons unable to judge because of their own meager experience.

In 1956 Safian (170) sounded a stern and timely warning about the fallacies then being promulgated by these nonplastic surgeons. He did not call this "the blind leading the blind," which he could have, but rather his article was entitled "Deceptive Concepts of Rhinoplasty." Dr. Safian began by saying, "I have pointed out that a rash of illogical procedures was being advocated by a group whose basic aim seems to have been to achieve headlines in medical literature. It appears that once these articles have appeared in print in some technical medical journal, the 'new' procedure is quietly dropped without retraction and is abandoned by its sponsors." His article was a sobering one, and is well worth reading today.

Back into the mainstream

Perhaps the most significant advance in the 1950s was the development of silicone rubber as an implant material. There were several scattered articles about its use for building up depressed or saddle noses, and the collective work was presented as a new chapter in the second revised printing of Brown and McDowell's *Plastic Surgery of the Nose* (23), which appeared in 1965.

During the last 15 years, evidence has been increasing that the "pay dirt" lode in the great mine of rhinoplastic information is nearly exhausted. The nose is a small organ with a rather simple anatomical structure; in two-thirds of a century, the fine investigative surgeons at work seem to have exhausted most of the possibilities for desirable structural changes in this small and simple organ. The situation is not unlike that which has existed for 50 years with regard to operations for indirect inguinal hernia.

There were, in the 1950s and 1960s, a number of articles published on new instruments for accomplishing old purposes. For example, Seltzer published a book entitled *Plastic Surgery of the Nose* (184) in 1949. During the next 5 years he also published 11 articles on assorted new rhinoplastic instruments; most of these did not catch the imagination of other surgeons. In 1957 his next-to-the-last article (entitled *The Rhinoplastic Surgeon and the Possibility of a Lawsuit*) (185) appeared. This was followed in 1960 by his final article *General Medical Practice and Corrective Rhinoplastic Surgery* (186). This dwindling output may have been due to age, health, or other personal reasons, of course—but it also came at a time when the possibilities of finding any new methods of merit for doing a rhinoplasty were dwindling.

During the 1960s and 1970s most of the articles published on rhinoplasty were "rehashes." Perhaps new were a few which advocated the trimming (or carving) of the alar cartilages by incisions made within, or through, the cartilages—rather than first separating the cartilages as anatomical units to obtain clear visibility of each entire unit before trimming it. There remains a considerable difference of opinion as to the value, or lack of value, in this approach. Some feel it is obfuscating; others point out that the published results are seldom as good as those published from the classic methods; others like it very much, saying that it is quicker and easier and exposure of each entire unit is not necessary.

In 1962 Hiebert and Brooks (71) republished an old and discarded method, developed in Germany, of inserting bone or cartilage grafts (or implants) into the nose by going through the mouth. They gave Schmid (177–179) prior credit for his 1952 and 1957 articles on the subject; in turn, Schmid gave Link (94) credit for his 1951 article. In actuality, the procedure is more ancient than that—but many surgeons believe the visibility is less and the possibility of infection is greater when one places transplants or implants through the mouth, rather than through a columellar incision.

There have been a few new and worthwhile developments in this region of diminishing returns, however. In 1967 Millard (136) described a method for thinning thick alae, one that was needed and which works. In 1963 Millard had described the use of chondromucosal flaps from the alae for relief of the retracted columella, or in reverse from the septum for relief of a notched or retracted alar margin; this was amplified in a 1972 article (138).

Dingman and Walter (45) described in 1969 the elongation of a short nose with composite grafts from the ear, a remarkable solution to a very difficult problem.

In 1971 Millard (137) described the bringing forward of both alae and the columella with three little composite grafts from the ear; this was an ingenious solution to the severe problem which exists when one tries to correct a mild congenital retrusion of the lower part of the nose.

Some books

The number of books on plastic surgery of the nose published since World War II has not been great. We have mentioned the 1952 edition (22) and the 1965 edition (23) of Brown and McDowell's book, and the 1949 Seltzer (184) book. J. W. Maliniac's book, *Rhinoplasty and Facial Contour* (115), was published in 1947 and reissued or republished in 1965. In 1957 a book by M. Aubry and J. C. Giraud, entitled *Chirurgie Fonctionelle, Correctrice et Restauratrice du Nez, La Rhinoplastie* (5), was published in the French language. In 1967 *Chirurgie Plastica del Naso* (52) by Filippi and Fruttero was published in the Italian language.

In 1967 also, Denecke and Meyer's extensive opus, *Corrective and Reconstructive Rhinoplasty* (42) appeared. This book probably represents the most complete miscellaneous compilation from the literature to that date. Unfortunately it gave equal prominence to currently used procedures that would work well and to antiquated, discarded procedures that would not work at all—with no especial recommendation (in most instances) for one over the other. The book was also distinguished by a total absence of any documented result by any operation—a most unusual stance for a work on esthetic surgery.

In 1972 Goldwyn's *Unfavorable Result in Plastic Surgery* (64) appeared, pointing out the problems that could occur in rhinoplastic and other esthetic surgery, and how to avoid them. Also there appeared in 1974 a beautifully printed book, *Cosmetic Facial Surgery* (158), by Rees and Wood-Smith. Later in 1973 John R. Lewis' excellent *Atlas of Aesthetic Plastic Surgery* (92) appeared. Finally, 1973 saw an exquisite reprinting of the Meiotti edition of that great classic *De Curturom Chirurgia per Insitionem*, written by Gaspare Tagliacozzi (198). The reprinted work was edited by F. Ortiz-Monasterio, of Mexico, D. F., Mexico.

Finale

With the above we end our recital of the history of rhinoplasty (119–133), and we append to it a brief, skeleton bibliography.

If any reader has a desire for more information, the author has compiled a complete bibliography (1,660 entries) of the world's literature (papers and books) on plastic surgery of the nose. This encompasses the period from 3,500 B.C. through 1973 A.D., and copies will be furnished at cost to those who request them.

Acknowledgment

Some of the earlier material in this review was published in the September 1952 issue of *Plastic and Reconstructive Surgery*, and is reproduced here by permission of the Williams & Wilkins Co.

References

1. Aldunate, E.: A new nasal osteotome. Plast. Reconstr. Surg. 4: 395, 1949.

2. Alves, O.: Costal graft and ivory inclusions in reconstruction of saddle nose. Rev. Otolaringol. São Paulo 4: 843, 1936.

3. Arkin, L.: A case of auto-transplantation of bone for nasal deformity due to syphilis. Boston Med. Surg. J. 172: 672, 1915.

4. Ashley, F.L., and King, E.D.: New type of metal nasal splint. Plast. Reconstr. Surg. 5: 536, 1950.

5. Aubry, M., and Giraud, J.C.: Chirurgie Fonctionelle, Correctrice, et Restauratrice du Nez. *La Rhinoplastie*. Librairie Arnette, Paris, 1956.

6. Aufricht, G.: Dental moulding compound cast and adhesive strapping in rhinoplasty. Arch. Otolaryngol. 32: 333, 1940.

7. Aufricht, G.: Hints and surgical details in rhinoplasty. Laryngoscope 53: 317, 1943.

8. Bames, H.O.: Elective rhinoplasty. Plast. Reconstr. Surg. 8: 113, 1951.

9. Barsky, A.J.: Moulded bone graft. Surgery 18: 755, 1945.

10. Becker, O.J.: Nasal speculum for rhinoplastic surgery. Plast. Reconstr. Surg. 3: 84, 1948.

11. Berger, P.: Rhinoplasty by the Italian method. Bull. Acad. Med. (Paris) 35: 204, 1896.

12. Berndorfer, A.: Importance of physiognomy in esthetic rhinoplasty. Plast. Reconstr. Surg. 6: 242, 1950.

13. Bigelow, H.J.: Periosteum of forehead transplanted in rhinoplastic operation; necrosis of skull. Boston Med. Surg. J. 76: 347, 1867.

14. Blair, V.P.: Total and subtotal restoration of the nose. J.A.M.A. 85: 1931, 1925.

15. Boyd, E., and Gaillie, W.E.: Restoration of nose by transferred flap including bone graft. Can. Med. Assoc. J. 8: 241, 1918.

16. Breasted, J.H.: Edwin Smith Surgical Papyrus, in Facsimile and Hieroglyphic with Translation and Commentary. University of Chicago Press, Chicago, 1930.

17. Brown, A.M.: Elephantiasis nostras nasalis. Plast. Reconstr. Surg. 6: 467, 1950.

18. Brown, J.B.: Preserved and fresh homotransplants of cartilage. Surg. Gynecol. Obstet. 70: 1079, 1940.

19. Brown, J.B.: Reconstructive surgery of the nose. In Nelson's Loose-Leaf System of Surgery 8: 237, 1940.

20. Brown, J.B., and Cannon, B.: Composite free grafts of skin and cartilage from ear. Surg. Gynecol. Obstet. 82: 253, 1946.

21. Brown, J.B., and DeMere, F.M.: Establishing a preserved cartilage bank. Plast. Reconstr. Surg. 3: 283, 1948.

22. Brown, J.B., and McDowell, F.: Plastic Surgery of the Nose. C.V. Mosby Co., St. Louis, 1951.

23. Brown, J.B. and McDowell, F.: Plastic Surgery of the Nose. Second Edition. Charles C. Thomas Co., Springfield, Ill. 1965.

24. Brunner, H.: Fate of autogenous rib cartilage transplanted into nose. Plast. Reconstr. Surg. 4: 439, 1949.

25. Buchanan, G.: Rhinoplasty from forehead, including periosteum in the flap. Lancet 2: 148, 1865.

26. Cardoso, A.D.: Reconstruction of cicatricial nasal retraction after leishmaniasis. Plast. Reconstr. Surg. 7: 309, 1951.

27. Carpue, J.C.: An Account of Two Successful Operations for Restoring a Lost Nose From the Integuments of the Forehead. London, Longman, 1816. Reprinted (in part), Plast. Reconstr. Surg. 44: 175, 1969.

28. Carter, W.W.: Cases of nasal deformity corrected by transplantation of bone. Med. Rec. 85: 237, 1914.

29. Carter, W.W.: Value and ultimate fate of bone and cartilage transplants in nasal deformities. Laryngoscope 33: 196, 1923.

30. Cinelli, A.A.: New instruments for use in rhinoplastic surgery. Arch. Otolaryngol. 32: 1102, 1940.

31. Cinelli, A.A.: Collapse of the nares. Arch. Otolaryngol. 33: 683, 1941.

32. Cohen, L.: Correction of saddle nose with mixed implants of bone and cartilage. Tr. Am. Laryngol. Rhinol. Otol. Soc. 33: 233, 1927.

33. Cohen, L.: Advantage of mixed bone and cartilage grafts in correction of saddle nose. Trans. Am. Laryngol. Rhinol. Otol. Soc. 46: 370, 1940.

34. Converse, J.M.: Corrective surgery of nasal tip. Ann. Otol. Rhinol. Laryngol. 49: 895, 1940.

35. Converse, J.M.: New forehead flap for reconstruction of nose. Proc. R. Soc. Med. 35: 811, 1942. Also J. Laryngol. Otol. 57: 508, 1942.

36. Converse, J.M.: Corrective surgery of nasal deviations. Arch. Otolaryngol. 52: 5, 1950.

37. Czerny: Three plastic operations. Gesell. Chir. 14: 212, 1895. Reprinted (in part), Plast. Reconstr. Surg. 45: 595, 1970.

38. Dahmann, H.: Cork as plastic material for correction of saddle nose. Z. Laryngol. Rhinol. 20: 451, 1931.

39. Daley, J.: Use of boiled cartilage as nasal implant. Eye, Ear, Nose Throat Mon. 26: 31, 1947.

40. Davis, W.B.: External nasal deformities and methods used in their repair. Arch. Otolaryngol. 36: 619, 1942.

41. DeKleine, E.H.: The chondrojet. Plast. Reconstr. Surg. 3: 95, 1948.

42. Denecke, J.H., and Meyer, R.: Plastic Surgery of the Head and Neck: Corrective and Reconstructive Rhinoplasty. Springer-Verlag, New York, Heidelberg, Berlin 1967.

43. Dieffenbach, J.F.: Die Operative Chirurgie. Leipzig, F.A. Brockhaus, 1845.

44. Dingman, R.O.: Repair of facial and cranial defects with iliac bone. Plast. Reconstr. Surg. 6: 179, 1950.

45. Dingman, R.O., and Walter, C.: Use of composite ear grafts in correction of the short nose. Plast. Reconstr. Surg. 43: 117, 1969.

46. Douglas, B.: Relief of vestibular nasal obstruction. Plast. Reconstr. Surg. 9: 42, 1952.

47. Dufourmentel, L.: Corrective Surgery of the Nose. Press of the Universities of France, Paris, 1926.

48. Dufourmentel, L., and Ginested: Acrylic inclusions for deformities; two cases of elimination of prosthesis. Mem. Acad. Chir. 74: 201, 1948.

49. Dupertuis, S.M.: Free ear lobe grafts of skin and fat; value in reconstruction about nostrils. Plast. Reconstr. Surg. 1: 135, 1946.

50. Dupertuis, S.M.: Growth of young human autogenous cartilage grafts. Plast. Reconstr. Surg. 5: 486, 1950.

51. Ellison, S.K.: Operation for depressed nose. Lancet 1: 394, 1894.

52. Filippi, B., and Fruterro, F.: Chirurgia Plastica del Naso. Sabatelli Editoria, Savona, Italy, 1967.

53. Finney, J.M.T.: Rhinoplasty by means of one of the fingers. Surg. Gynecol. Obstet. 5: 23, 1907.

54. Fomon, S. et al: Physiological principles in rhinoplasty. Arch. Otolaryngol. 53: 3, 1951.

55. Fred, G.B.: Nasal tip in rhinoplasty; invaginating technic to prevent secondary dropping. Ann. Otol. Rhinol. Laryngol. 59: 215, 1950.

56. Gatewood, W.L.: Substitution of chisel for saw in reconstructive surgery of nose. Plast. Reconstr. Surg. 2: 149, 1947.

57. Gerrie, J., Cloutier, G.E., and Woolhouse, F.M.: Carved cancellous bone grafts in rhinoplasty. Plast. Reconstr. Surg. 6: 196, 1950.

58. Gersuny: Hard-paraffin prosthesis. Zentralbl. Chir. 1: 86, 1903.

59. Gillies, H.: Plastic Surgery of the Face. H. Frowde, Hodder, and Stoughton Co., London, 1920.

60. Gillies, H.: Deformities of the syphilitic nose. Br. Med. J., 2: 977, 1923.

61. Gillies, H.: New free graft (of skin and ear cartilage) applied to reconstruction of nostril. Br. J. Surg. 30: 305, 1943.

62. Gillies, H., and Kristensen, H.K.: Ox cartilage in plastic surgery. Br. J. Plast. Surg. 4: 64, 1951.

63. Gnudi, M.T., and Webster, J.P.: Life and Times of Gaspare Tagliacozzi. Herbert Reichner, New York, 1950.

64. Goldwyn, R.M.: The Unfavorable Result in Plastic Surgery. Little, Brown & Co., Boston, 1972.

65. Gonzales-Ulloa, M.: Use of bone from cattle in restoration of saddle nose. Arq. Clin. Cir. Exp. 6: 535, 1942.

66. Grasch, F.M.: Correction of saddle nose with synthetic acrylic resin. An. Med. Barcelona 35: 340, 1948.

67. Greeley, P.W.: Nasal deformities, abrasions, and accidental tattoos, scars, keloids, and scar contractures. Surg. Clin. North Am. 22: 253, 1943.

68. Hardie, J.: On a new rhinoplastic operation. Br. Med. J. p. 393, 1875.

69. Herbert, J.G.: Another external nasal splint. Plast. Reconstr. Surg. 2: 159, 1947.

70. Heinberg, C.J.: Modern aspects of rhinoplasty. Laryngoscope 69: 789, 1959.

71. Hiebert, A.E., and Brooks, H.W.: Sublabial approach for the insertion of L-shaped bone strut for the correction of saddle nose. Plast. Reconstr. Surg. 29: 608, 1962.

72. Holt, J.A.B., and Lloyd, R.S.: Rhinoplasty: use of methyl methacrylate implants. Arch. Otolaryngol. 47: 406, 1948.

73. Israel, J.: Two methods of rhinoplasty. Arch. Klin. Chir. 53: 255, 1896. Translation published in Plast. Reconstr. Surg. 46: 80, 1970.

74. Joseph, J. Operative reduction of the size of a nose (rhinomiosis). Berl. Klin. Wochenschr. 40: 882, 1898.

75. Joseph, J.: About some further nasal reductions. Berl. Klin. Wochenschr. p. 851, 1902.

76. Joseph, J.: Intranasal hump removal. Berl. Klin. Wochenschr. 30: 650, 1904.

77. Joseph, J.: Nasal reductions. Dtsche. Med. Wochenschr. 30: 1095, 1904. Translation published in Plast. Reconstr. Surg., 47: 79, 1971.

78. Joseph, J.: More about nasal reductions. Münch. Med. Wochenschr. 52: 1489, 1905.

79. Joseph, J.: Treatise on rhinoplasty. Berl. Klin. Wochenschr. 44: 470, 1907.

80. Joseph, J.: Correction of twisted nose. Dtsche. Med. Wochenschr. 49: 203, 1907.

81. Joseph, J.: Chapter on corrective nasal plastic. In Handbuch der Speziellen Chirurgie (edited by Katz and Blumenfeld). Leipzig, C. Kabitsch, 1922.

82. Joseph, J.: Nasal Plastic and Various Face Plastics, as well as Mammaplasty. Leipzig. C. Kabitsch, 1931.

83. Kazanjian, V.H.: Nasal deformities of syphilitic origin. Plast. Reconstr. Surg. 3: 517, 1948.

84. Keegan, D.F.: Rhinoplastic Operations, With a Description of Recent Improvements in the Indian Method. Ballière, Tindall, and Cox, London, 1900.

85. Kimball, G.H., and Drummond, N.R.: Vitallium for skeleton support. J. Oklahoma Med. Assoc. 34: 9, 1941.

86. Koechlin, H.: New instruments in rhinoplasty. Plast. Reconstr. Surg. 8: 132, 1951.

87. König, F.: A new method of correcting sunken noses with a skin-periosteal-bone forehead flap. Arch. Klin. Chir. 34: 165, 1886.

88. König, F.: On filling defects of the nostril wall. Berl. Klin. Wochenschr. 39: 137, 1902.

89. Küster, E.: Rhinoplasty from the arm. Arch. Klin. Chir. 48: 179, 1894.

90. Lamont, E.S.: Reconstructive surgery of the nose in congenital deformity, injury, and disease. Am. J. Surg. 65: 17, 1944.

91. Levy, R.: Rhinoplasty for saddlenose with bone transplantation from the tibia. Berl. Klin. Wochenschr. 47: 1557, 1910.

92. Lewis, J.R.: Atlas of Aesthetic Surgery. Little, Brown & Co., Boston, 1973.

93. Linhares, F.: Corrections of saddle nose by inclusion of Vitallium. Rev. Brasil. Cir. 14: 159, 1945. Ibid. 15: 449, 1946.

94. Link, R.: Plastic surgery of the cartilaginous framework of the nose. Z. Laryngol. 33: 74, 1951.

95. MacCollum, S.W.: Use of iliac bone in elevation of bridge of nose. Surgery 12: 97, 1942.

96. MacMillan, W.: Multiple knife for dicing cartilage. Plast. Reconstr. Surg. 3: 226, 1948.

97. Malbec, E.F.: Ivory prosthesis in partial rhinoplasty. Sem. Med. 1: 1374, 1938.

98. Malbec, E.F.: Partial rhinoplasty using marble prosthesis. Sem. Med. 2: 1173, 1940.

99. Malbec, E.F.: Osseous transplantations in partial rhinoplasties. Sem. Med. 2: 350, 1941.

100. Malbec, E.F.: Duraluminum in plastic surgery. Sem. Med. 1: 1016, 1941.

101. Malbec, E.F.: Bone autografts in partial rhinoplasties. Arq. Cir. Clin. Exp. 6: 163, 1942.

102. Malbec, E.F.: Osteocartilaginous homogenous grafts in partial rhinoplasties. Dia. Med. 15: 644, 1943.

103. Malbec, E.F.: Saddle nose; correction by means of tantalum prosthesis. Rev. Assoc. Med. Argent. 60: 361,1946.

104. Malbec, E.F.: Preserved cartilage in corrective rhinoplasty. Dia. Med. 19: 1414, 1947. Also in Cong. Lat. Am. Cir. Plast. 1949.

105. Maliniac, J.W.: Comparative study of ivory and organic transplants in rhinoplasty. Laryngoscope 34: 883, 1924.

106. Maliniac, J.W.: Use of ivory in rhinoplasty. Arch. Otolaryngol. 1: 599, 1925.

107. Maliniac, J.W.: Nasal deformities, their prevention and correction following submucous resection. Arch. Otolaryngol. 6: 320, 1927.

108. Maliniac, J.W.: Plastic and reconstructive procedures. N.Y. Med. J. 28: 6, 1928.

109. Maliniac, J.W.: Rhinoplasty; a few statistical data. Eye, Ear, Nose Throat Mon. 9: 194, 1930.

110. Maliniac, J.W.: Rhinophyma. Arch. Otolaryngol. 13: 270, 1931.

111. Maliniac, J.W.: Correction of depressions by transposition of lateral cartilages. Arch. Otolaryngol. 15: 280, 1932.

112. Maliniac, J.W.: Cartilage and ivory; indications and contraindications for use as nasal support. Arch. Otolaryngol. 17: 649, 1933.

113. Maliniac, J.W.: Prevention of late sequelae in corrective rhinoplasty. Am. J. Surg. 50: 84, 1940.

114. Maliniac, J.W.: Procedure for elevation of nasal dorsum by transposition of lateral cartilages. Arch. Otolaryngol. 41: 214, 1945.

115. Maliniac, J.W.: Rhinoplasty and Restoration of Facial Contour. F.A. Davis Co., Philadelphia, 1947.

116. Mangoldt, F. von: Reconstruction of saddle nose by cartilage overlay. Gesell. Chir. 29: 460, 1900. Translation published in Plast. Reconstr. Surg. 46: 495, 1970.

117. Martin, B.C.: Cancellous bone grafts for restoration of contour. Plast. Reconstr. Surg. 3: 202, 1948.

118. May, H.: The Rethi incision in rhinoplasty. Plast. Reconstr. Surg. 8: 123, 1951.

119. McDowell, F.: Kiel bone grafts. Plast. Reconstr. Surg. 41: 370, 1968.

120. McDowell, F.: Commentary on the Edwin Smith Surgical Papyrus. Plast. Reconstr. Surg. 43: 409, 1969.

121. McDowell, F.: Sushruta's ancient earlobe and rhinoplastic operations in India. Plast. Reconstr. Surg. 43: 517, 1969.

122. McDowell, F.: Development of plastic surgery from ancient times to the eighteenth century. Plast. Reconstr. Surg. 43: 618, 1969.

123. McDowell, F.: "The B.L. Bombshell" Plast. Reconstr. Surg. 44: 71, 1969.

124. McDowell, F.: Commentary on Bunger's paper. Plast. Reconstr. Surg. 44: 489, 1969.

125. McDowell, F.: Editorial addendum to Roe's paper. Plast. Reconstr. Surg. 45: 287, 1970.

126. McDowell, F.: Commentary on Weir's paper. Plast. Reconstr. Surg. 45: 390, 1970.

127. McDowell, F.: Commentary on the first free bone graft to the nose. Plast. Reconstr. Surg. 46: 83, 1970.

128. McDowell, F.: Commentary on the first cartilage graft to the nose. Plast. Reconstr. Surg. 46: 500, 1970.

129. McDowell, F.: Commentary on Joseph's paper. Plast. Reconstr. Surg. 47: 81, 1971.

130. McDowell, F.: Case of the elusive Mr. Lucas, the mysterious Major Heitland et al. Plast. Reconstr. Surg. 49: 77, 1972.

131. McDowell, F., Brown, J.B., and Fryer, M.P.: Surgery of the Face, Mouth, and Jaws. C.V. Mosby Co., St. Louis, 1954.

132. McDowell, F., and Enna, C.D.: Surgical Rehabilitation in Leprosy. Williams & Wilkins Co., Baltimore, 1974.

133. McDowell, F., Valone, J.A. and Brown, J.B.: Bibliography and historical note on plastic surgery of the nose. Plast. Reconstr. Surg. 10: 149, 1952.

134. McIndoe, A.H.: Restoration of depressed nose by grafting of cartilage; 6 cases. Proc. R. Soc. Med. 27: 1278, 1934.

135. Metzenbaum, M.: Recent fractures of the nose. Arch. Otolaryngol. 34: 723, 1941.

136. Millard, D.R.: Alar margin sculpturing. Plast. Reconstr. Surg. 40: 337, 1967.

137. Millard, D.R.: Congenital nasal tip retrusion and three little composite ear grafts. Case report. Plast. Reconstr. Surg. 48: 501, 1971.

138. Millard, D.R.: Versatility of a chondromucosal flap in the nasal vestibule. Plast. Reconstr. Surg. 50: 580, 1972.

139. Monks, G.H.: Correction, by operation, of some nasal deformities and disfigurements. Boston Med. Surg. J. 139: 262, 1898. Reprinted in Plast. Reconstr. Surg. 48: 485, 1971.

140. Morestin, H.: Depression and perforation of the wall of the nose; correction by autoplasty and graft of a strip of cartilage. Bull. Mem. Soc. Chir. Paris 40: 1194, 1914.

141. Mowlem, R.: Use and behavior of iliac bone grafts in restoration of nasal contour. Rev. Chir. Structive 8: 23, 1938.

142. Mowlem, R.: Iliac bone and cartilage transplants; use and behavior. Br. J. Surg. 29: 182, 1941.

143. Nelaton, Ch.: On a new procedure of rhinoplasty. Bull. Mem. Soc. Chir. Paris 26: 663, 1900.

144. Nelaton, Ch., and Ombredanne, L.: The Rhinoplasty. G. Steinheil C., Paris, 1904.

145. New, G.B.: Sickle flap for reconstruction of nose. Surg. Gynecol. Obstet. 80: 497, 1945.

146. New, G.B., and Austin, G.W.: The chrondrotome-ejector for shredding and inserting cartilage. Plast. Reconstr. Surg. 5: 444, 1950.

147. New, G.B.: and Erich, J.B.: Method to prevent fresh costal cartilage from warping. Am. J. Surg. 54: 435, 1941.

148. O'Connor, G.B., and Pierce, G.W.: Refrigerated cartilage isografts. Surg. Gynecol. Obstet. 67: 796, 1938.

149. Ollier: Osteoplasty applied to restoration of the nose. Gaz. Hop. Paris, P. 349, 1864.

150. Parsons, H.H.: A plaster nasal splint. Mil. Surg. 91: 212, 1942.

151. Peer, L.A.: Diced cartilage grafts. Arch. Otolaryngol. 38: 156, 1943.

152. Peer, L.A.: Cartilage grafting. S. Clin. North Am. 24: 408, 1944.

153. Peer, L.A.: Neglected cartilage graft (with experimental observation on growth of human cartilage grafts). Arch. Otolaryngol. 42: 384, 1945.

154. Pelliciari, D.D.: Columella and tip reconstruction. Plast. Reconstr. Surg. 4:98, 1949.

155. Penn, J., Jankowitz, J., and Bruwer, A.: Grated cadaver cartilage. Plast. Reconstr. Surg. 3: 228, 1948.

156. Prudente, A.: Surgical correction of uncomplicated saddle nose by partial inclusion of ivory. Rev. Assoc. Paulista Med. 5: 75, 1934.

157. Rapin, M.: Eight years' experience with synthetic acrylic resins in rhinoplasty. Pract. Otorhinolaryngol. 11: 425, 1949.

158. Rees, T.H., and Wood-Smith, D.: Cosmetic Surgery. W.B. Saunders Co., Phila. 1974.

159. Rethi, A.: Right and wrong in rhinoplastic surgery. Plast. Reconstr. Surg. 3: 361, 1948.

160. Roberts, G.: Management of nasal fractures. Laryngoscope 60: 557, 1950.

161. Roberts, J.B.: Suggestions for operative correction of syphilitic and other deformities of nose. Ann. Surg. 51: 173, 1910.

162. Roe., J.O.: The deformity termed pug nose and its correction by a simple operation. Med. Rec. 31: 621, 1887. Reprinted in Plast. Reconstr. Surg. 45: 78, 1970.

163. Roe, J.O.: The correction of angular deformities of the nose by a subcutaneous operation. Med. Rec. 40: 57, 1891. Reprinted in Plast. Reconstr. Surg. 45: 283, 1970.

164. Rotkitski, V.M.: Free bony, cartilaginous, and cutaneous rhinoplastic surgery. Khir. Arkh. Velyaminova 30: 431, 1914.

165. Rubin, L.R.: New rhinoplastic instrument. Plast. Reconstr. Surg. 3: 86, 1948.

166. Rubin, L.R.: Polyethelene—three year study. Plast. Reconstr. Surg. 7: 131, 1951.

167. Rubin, L.R., Robertson, G.W., and Shapiro, R.H.: Use of polyethylene in reconstructive surgery. Plast. Reconstr. Surg. 3: 5, 1948.

168. Safian, J.: Corrective Rhinoplastic Surgery. Paul Hoeber Co., New York, 1935.

169. Safian, J.: Failures in rhinoplastic surgery; causes and prevention. Am. J. Surg. 50: 274, 1940.

170. Safian, J.: Deceptive concepts of rhinoplasty. Plast. Reconstr. Surg. 18: 127, 1956.

171. Salinger, S.: Ivory implants for saddle nose; results in 50 cases. Ann. Otol. Rhinol. Laryngol. 40: 801, 1931.

172. Salinger, S.: Saddle nose; ivory and cartilage transplants. Illinois Med. J. 72: 412, 1937.

173. Salinger, S.: Injuries to nose in children. Arch. Otolaryngol. 34: 936, 1941.

174. Salinger, S.: Traumatic deformities of the nasal septum. Ann. Otol. Rhinol. Laryngol. 53: 274, 1944.

175. Scher, S.L.: The deformed nose. Arch. Otolaryngol. 34: 307, 1941.

176. Schilling: Rhjnoplasty with bone transplant. Krist. Kirurg. Forh., p. 42, 1915.

177. Schmid, E.: New methods for plastic surgery of nose. Beitr. Klin. Chir. 184: 385, 1952.

178. Schmid, E.: Nasal prostheses. Arch. Klin. Chir. 287: 736, 1957.

179. Schmid, E.: Reconstruction of shrunken nose by free transplantation. Dtsche. Zahn-, Mund-, Kieferheilk. 47: 339, 1966.

180. Sedillot: New procedure and observations in rhinoplasty. Gaz. Med. Strasbourg 16: 269, 1856.

181. Seeley, R.C.: Reconstruction of nasal tip; new technic. Plast. Reconstr. Surg. 3: 594, 1948.

182. Seltzer, A.P.: Improved method for narrowing the nose. Ann. Otol. Rhinol. Laryngol. 52: 640, 1943.

183. Seltzer, A.P.: Plastic repair of the deviated septum associated with deflected tip. Arch. Otolaryngol. 40: 433, 1944.

184. Seltzer, A.P.: Plastic Surgery of the Nose. J.B. Lippincott Co., Philadelphia, 1949.

185. Seltzer, A.P.: The rhinoplastic surgeon and the possibility of a lawsuit. Ann. Otol. Rhinol. Laryngol. 66: 208, 1957.

186. Seltzer, A.P.: General medical practice and corrective nasal surgery. Am. Pract. 11: 177, 1960.

187. Sheehan, J.E.: Plastic Surgery of the Nose. Paul Hoeber Co., New York, First Edition 1925, Second Edition, 1936.

188. Spanier, F.: Alloplastic and heteroplastic grafts in reconstruction of facial defects, especially saddle nose; use of ivory. Rev. Chir. Structive p. 391, 1936.

189. Steffensen, W.H.: Reconstruction of nasal septum. Plast. Reconstr. Surg. 2: 66, 1947.

190. Steinthal, K: Rhinoplasty from chest skin. Beitr. Klin. Chir. 29: 485, 1900.

191. Stout, P.S.: Bovine cartilage in correction of deformities. Laryngoscope 43: 976, 1933.

192. Straatsma, C.R.: Problems in nasal plastic surgery. Laryngoscope 50: 1092, 1940.

193. Straith, C.L.: A method of rhinoplasty. Rev. Chir. Plastique 3: 109, 1933.

194. Straith, C.L.: Elongation of nasal columella; new operative technic. Plast. Reconstr. Surg. 1: 79, 1946.

195. Straith, C.L., and Slaughter, W.B.: Grafts of preserved cartilage in restoration of facial contour. J.A.M.A. 116: 2008, 1941.

196. Sushruta Samhita: Ancient earlobe and rhinoplastic operations in India. Reprinted in Plast. Reconstr. Surg. 43: 515, 1969.

197. Symanowski, J. von: Handbuch der Operativen Chirurgie. Vieweg u. Sohn, Braunschweig, 1870.

198. Tagliacozzi, G.: De Curtorum Chirurgia Per Insitionem, etc., Venice, Gaspar Bindonus Jr., 1597. Facsimile publication of the Meiotti Edition (edited and foreword by Fernando Ortiz-Monasterio, M.D.), Libreria Manuel Porrua, S.A., Mexico, D.F., Mexico, 1973.

199. Tamerin, J.A.: A method for reconstruction of a large nasal fistula. Plast. Reconstr. Surg. 7: 157, 1951.

200. Thiersch, K.V.: A rhinoplastic modification. Gesell. Chir. 8: 67, 1879.

201. Vadala, A.J., and Somers, K.: Preserved homogenous cancellous bone for rhinoplasty. Mil. Surg. 107: 281, 1950.

113

202. Vaillancourt, J.: Cartilage transplantation in a case of deformity of the nose. Bull. Med. Quebec 15: 194, 1913.

203. Warren, J.M.: Rhinoplastic operation. Boston Med. Surg. J. 16: 69, 1837.

204. Webster, J.P., and Deming, E.G.: Surgical treatment of bifid nose. Plast. Reconstr. Surg. 6: 1, 1950.

205. Weir, R.F.: On restoring sunken noses. N.Y.M.J. 56: 449, 1892. Reprinted in Plast. Reconstr. Surg. 45: 382, 1970.

206. Wible, L.E., Trombetta, A., and Wineinger, G.E.: Use of tantalum screen in repair of nasal deformities. U.S. Armed Forces Med. J. 2: 653, 1951.

207. Wolfe, M.M.: Technic of ivory implant for correction of saddle nose. Arch. Surg. 37: 800, 1938.

208. Young, F.: Principle to be considered in transplanting costal cartilage for repairing deficiencies of nasal skeleton. Ann. Surg. 108: 670, 1946.

209. Young, F.: Surgical repair of nasal deformities. Plast. Reconstr. Surg. 4: 59, 1949.

210. Zeno, L.: Marble prosthesis in correction of saddle nose. An. Cir. 5: 111, 1939.

Aesthetic Plastic Surgery 2:75–94, 1978

History of the Aesthetic Surgery of the Ear

Jack E. Davis M.D. with the assistance of
Horacio H. Hernandez M.D.
Buenos Aires, Argentina

Aesthetics is a relative term. The concept of beauty with regard to the ear has changed with time and place. Buddhas have been modeled, and the monoliths of aristocrats of Easter Island with enormous ears as a sign of distinction. The old Inca guards of honor were the *orejones*. Captain Cook (33) described natives of New Guinea carrying knives in their earlobes. Prominent ears are a sign of success and opulence in Japan today. The organ has served to hang varied ornaments. From the most ancient times personality traits have been attributed to ear shape. The clay tablets of the great library of Ashurbanipal (about 650 B.C.), unearthed in Nineveh, Assyria, told that the shape of the ears of a newborn foretold his future character (73). At the close of the last century, Lombroso's legal medical treatise (77) even described the "congenital criminal" from ear characteristics.

The roots of aesthetic and reconstructive surgery of the ear are closely entwined, and the dividing line is arbitrary. Academically, change of shape and/or reduction in size has been considered aesthetic, but increase in size means adding tissue and is therefore reconstructive.

Ear repair was first mentioned in the Vedas (knowledge, sacred lore) from ancient India, where Sushruta, a disciple of Dhanvantarti, wrote his encyclopedic ayurvedic medical treatise, which has been called the Sanhitas. The date is uncertain, but the style seems to indicate that it was written about 600 B.C., which means it was contemporary with Buddha. As oral transmission of knowledge had existed for many centuries, these writings are the product of experience long before. There was little knowledge of anatomy because at that time to dissect the dead was defiling. Surgeons of the time used 101 steel instruments, which were kept in a wooden box. Anesthesia was with alcohol. Postoperatively, patients were allowed a special diet of meat, normally forbidden for Hindus. Repair for an earlobe with cheek flaps is described in the sixteenth section of the book on surgery, the *Uttara Sthana*. Little progress was added to these classic writings for the next 25 centuries in India, where this surgery remained in the hands of the potter caste (3, 12, 41, 77, 84, 86, 111, 112, 134).

Plastic surgery of the ear is not mentioned in the Edwin Smith or Ebers papyruses of ancient Egypt. The outstanding surgical work of Hua T'o in China was lost when he

---

Address reprint requests to Jack E. Davis, M.D., Sarandi 182, Buenos Aires, Argentina

0364-216X/0002–0075 $04.00
© 1978 Springer-Verlag New York Inc.

115

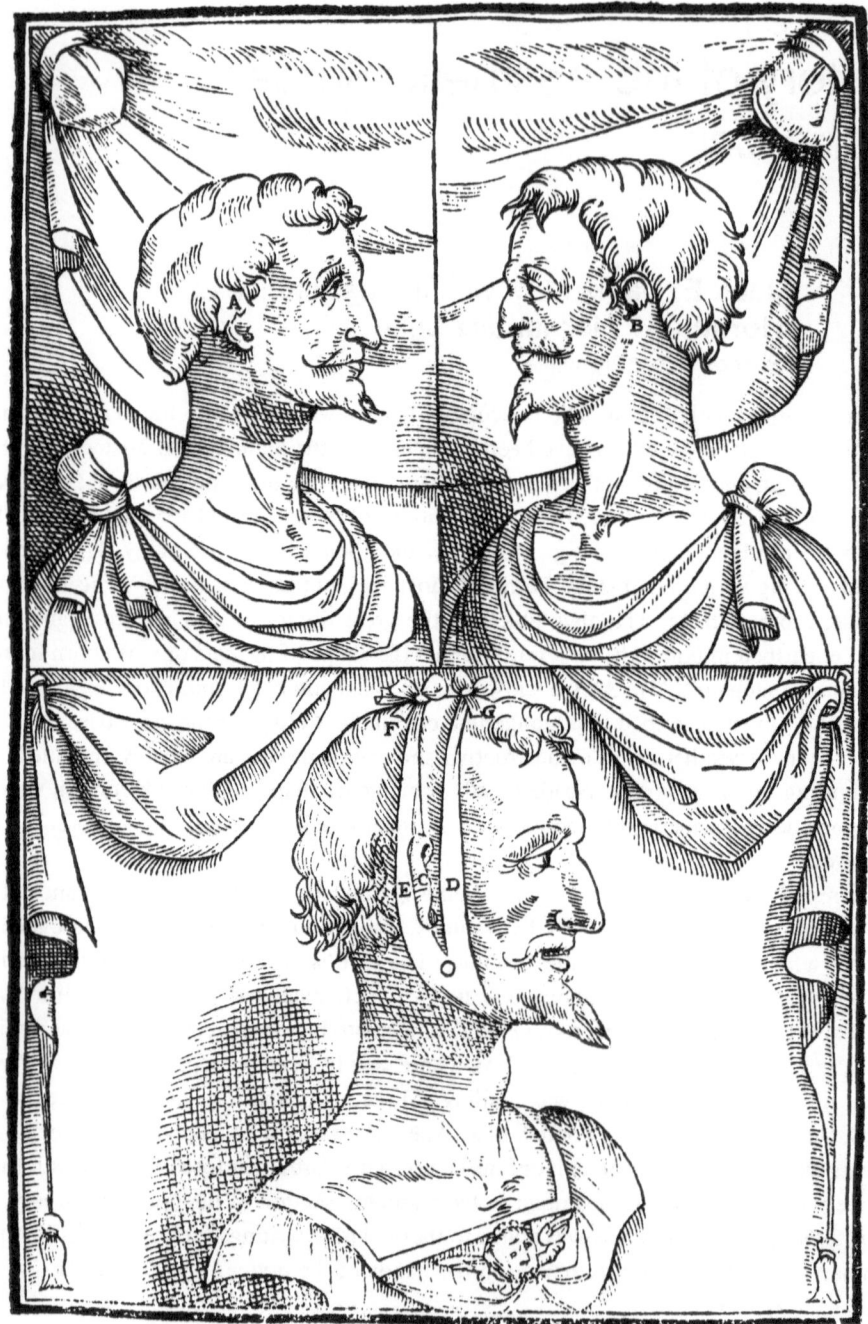

Fig. 1A and **B.** Reconstruction of the upper and lower halves of the ear. From *De Curtorum Chirurgia*, by Gaspare Tagliacozzi, 1597.

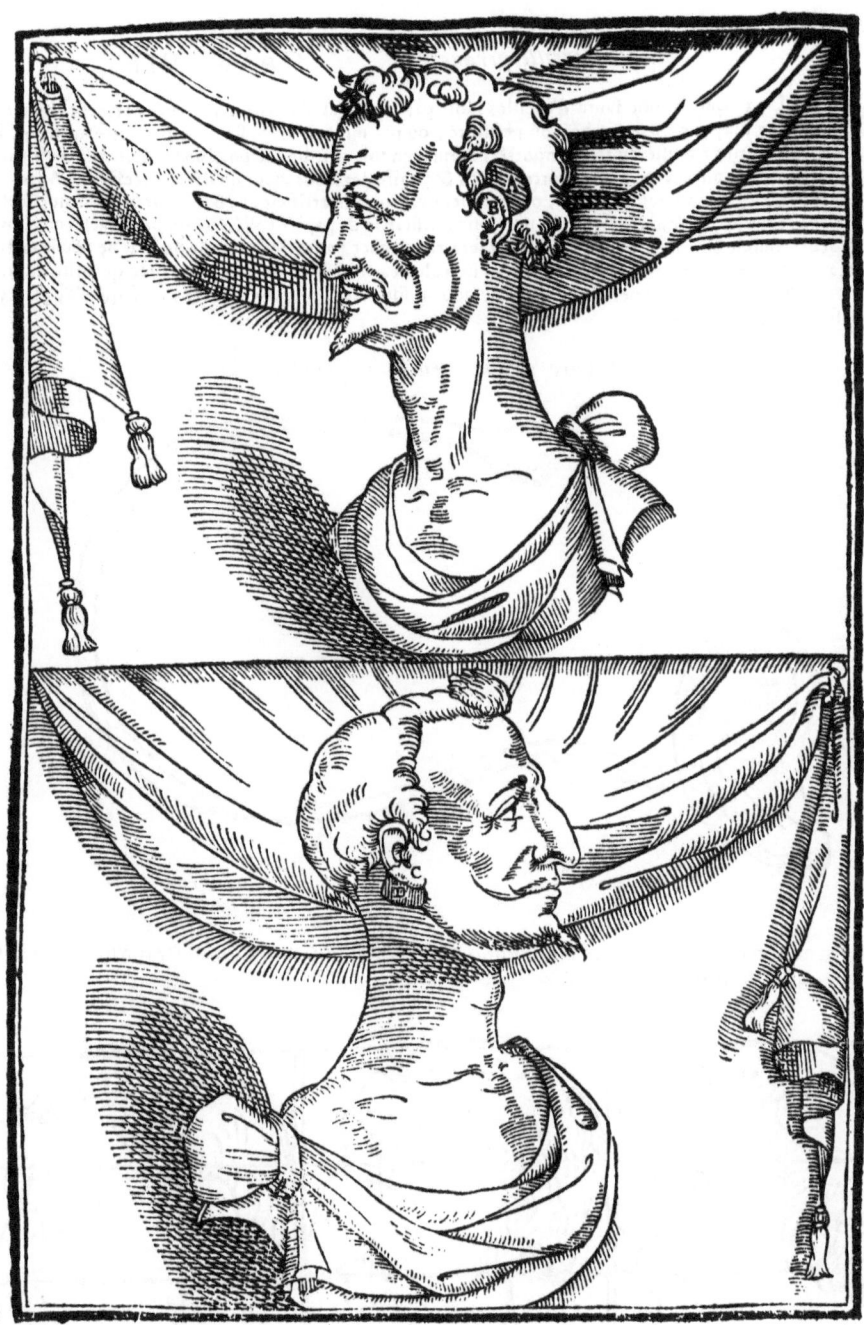

De l'oreille perduë.   Cʜᴀᴘ. VII.

Evx qui auront faute d'oreilles, foit par le defaut de nature, ou par accident, comme par playe, ou par vn charbon peftiferé, ou par morfure de befte, ou par autre maniere, fi l'oreille n'a efté du tout emporté, & qu'il en foit refte bonne portion on doit trouuer le cartilage auec vne perite porte-piece, & y faire des trous, tant qu'ilfera neceffaire. Apres la cicatrifation defdits trous, on attachera vne oreille artificielle : & où l'oreille auroit efté du tout amputee,on y en appliquera vne artificielle de papier collé,ou cuir boüilly, façonnée de bonne grace, comme tu vois par cette figure. Et fera tenuë auec petits liens autour de la tefte : où le malade laiftera croiftre fes cheueux longs,ou portera vne calotte. Auffi lors qu'il y a eu grande quantité du crane perdu, faudra porter vn bonnet de cuir boüilly pour refifter aux iniures externes, ainfi que i'ay par cy-deuant efcrit aux playes de teftes.

Figure d'vne oreille artificielle.

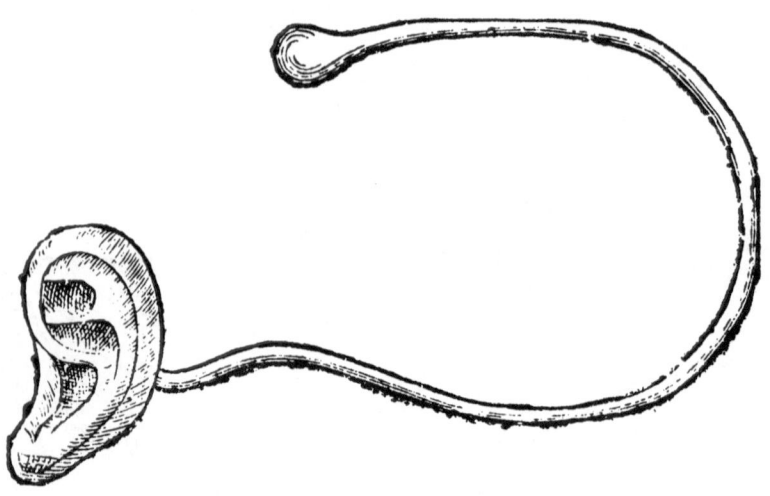

De

Fig. 2. An ear prosthesis made of enamelled metal, attached to the head by a wire hoop. From *Les Oeuvres d'Ambroise Paré,* 1652.

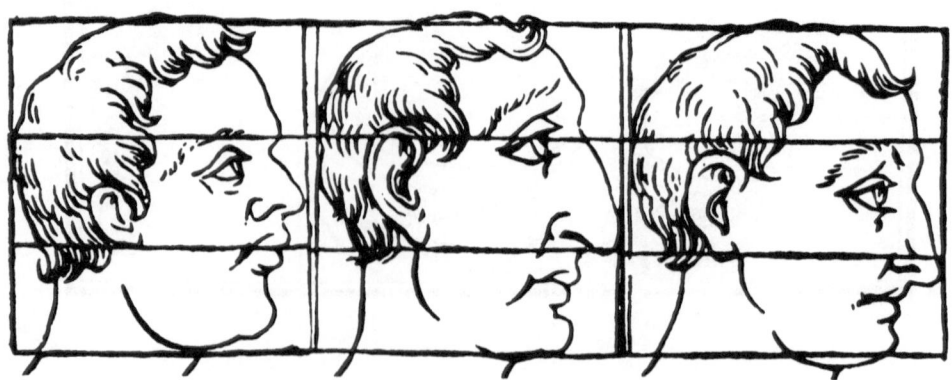

Fig. 3. Studies of various ear shapes; the "ideal" ear in the (right) drawing. From *Della Fisionomia dell'Huomo,* by Giambattista della Porta, 1623.

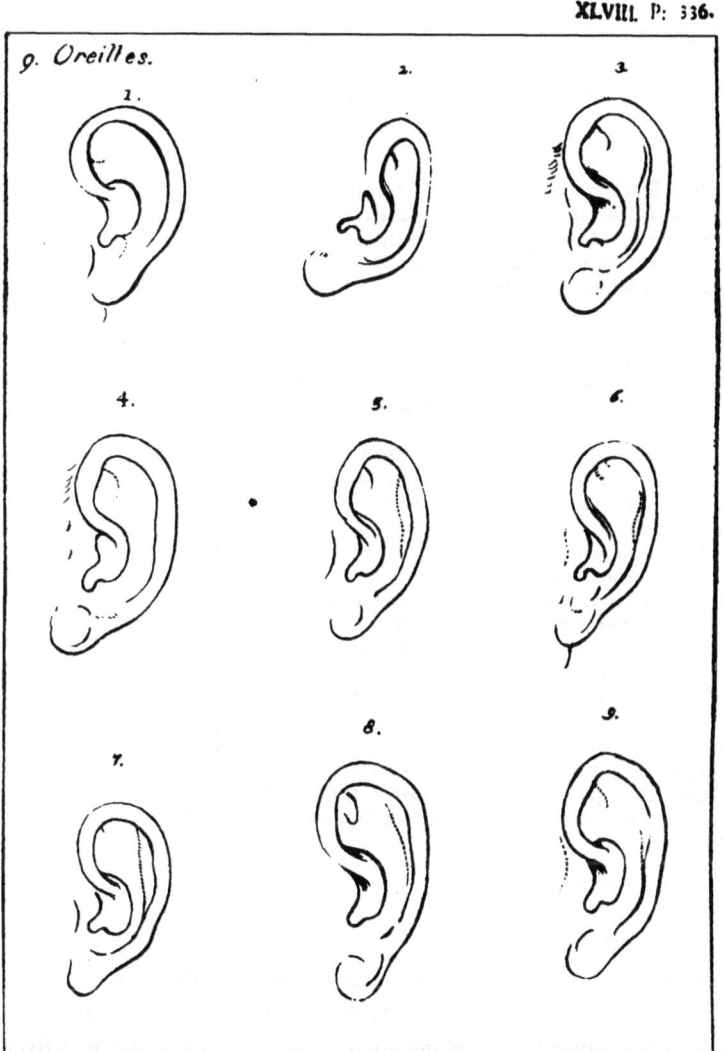

Fig. 4A–4D. Lavater's physiognomic studies of ear shapes. From *Essai sur la Physionomie,* by J. G. Lavater, 1783.

burned his memoirs in his cell before his execution. Nothing is found in the writing of Hippocrates of Greece. From the Chin dynasty (229–351 A.D.) and Fang Kan of the Tang dynasty (618–901 A.D.) in China, only plastic surgery of the lips is referred to (84, 86, 89, 111, 112).

But the teachings of Erasistratos (Island of Kios) and Herophilus (Alexandria) were collected by the great historian of medicine Aulus Cornelius Celsus (about 30 A.D.). Although it is doubtful that he was a practicing physician, he wrote a classic textbook on medicine that was used for many centuries. In books VII and VIII, Celsus referred to repair of mutilated ears with advancement quadrangle flaps. He mentioned that projecting

336 CINQUIEME FRAGM. DES DIFFÉRENTES PARTIES DU CORPS.

A D D I T I O N A.

9. OREILLES.

Puisque je fuis encore fi peu avancé dans l'étude de l'oreille, il me fera difficile de commenter d'une manière politive & fatisfaifante les Additions que je fais à ce Chapitre. La comparaifon des extrêmes me fournira avec le temps des inductions plus certaines, cependant je ne crois rien rifquer en affurant que parmi les deffins de la Planche ci-jointe, il ne s'en trouve pas un feul qui caractérife l'imbécillité.

L'oreille 1 me paroît la plus délicate, la plus foible.

La 2de. eft plus fine, plus attentive & plus réflèchie.

La 3e l'emporte fur la 1re à l'égard de l'activité & de l'énergie. J'y entrevois un génie productif, riche en talens, & particulièrement doué de celui de l'éloquence.

J'adopte à peu près la même définition pour le N° 4. mais avec quelques modifications, dont je cherche la raifon dans la partie du haut. D'un autre côté le contour ferpenté qui borde l'enfoncement, pourroit bien être le figne de la bonhommie.

5 eft de beaucoup plus foible & plus borné que 2, 3, 4.

6 eft encore plus uni & moins nuancé. J'excepte pourtant la pointe qui eft au deffous de l'enfoncement, & qui, en dépit de la médiocrité des facultés, femble indiquer un talent particulier, j'ignore lequel?

Suivant mon texte, l'oreille 7 annonce un homme modefte, humble & doux, peut-être timide & craintif.

Le 8, & encore moins le 9, ne fauroient convenir à des efprits ordinaires.

Il feroit intéreffant de rapprocher une centaine de têtes différentes & connues, & d'abftraire en conféquence le caractère propre & fpécifique de leurs oreilles. Dans celles que nous avons ici devant nous, le bout eft dégagé; ce qu'on peut toujours regarder comme un bon augure pour les facultés intellectuelles.

PLANCHE XLVIII.

4B

cartilage should be removed and insisted on a particular type of healing. Also, he explained how to make an ear canal for atresia by trephining the mastoid and placing a wooden peg in the hole until healing by second intention took place. Paul of Aeginus lived in Alexandria in the seventh century A.D., and his works were translated into Arabic. Thus he is known after the great fire destroyed the famous library. In his volume on surgery, book VIII, microtia is classified as congenital and traumatic. In Arabic surgery, only Rhazes (about 900 A.D.) discussed repair of mutilated ears with the same methods of Celsus and Paul (41, 84, 86, 111, 112, 134).

From there, our historical information jumps to the Renaissance, when a center of surgery was in Palermo, Sicily, in the sixteenth century. The two Brancas, father and son, worked in secret at Catania. Antonio, the son, seems to have used arm flaps to repair the lips and ears. Their work is known from only a few letters of visitors and patients of that time, and reference to the ears is by Bartolomeo Facio, historian of Alfonso I, of Aragon and Naples (134).

XLIX. P: 337.

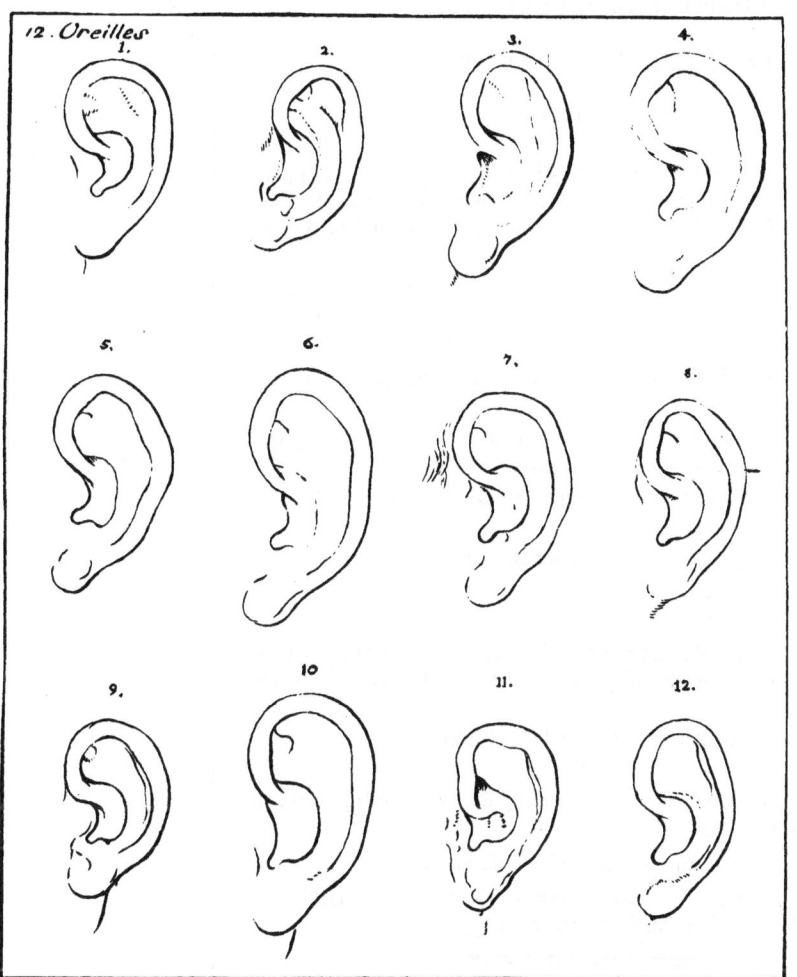

4C

Without a doubt, the most scholarly and detailed description with a clear technique in ear repair is found in Gaspari Tagliacozzi's *De Curtorum Chirurgia*, which was written toward the end of the sixteenth century. He described and beautifully illustrated reconstruction of the upper and lower halves of the ear (Fig. 1). Local skin flaps were used, bent over on themselves, leaving the defect to close by second intention. Modern methods have only added a skin graft to cover the defect for repair of the lobule (Converse). One of Tagliacozzi's disciples, Giovanne Cortesi, made a point that is still significant today: it is easier to reconstruct the lower half of the ear than the upper. Tagliacozzi was a distinguished teacher of anatomy and surgery at the University of Bologna, Italy. He was buried in the monastery of San Giovanni Battista but was disinterred by the nuns because they heard strange noises that they attributed to him with religious superstition at the time of the

121

CHAPITRE IX. des OREILLES.   337

A   D   D   I   T   I   O   N   B.

12. Oreilles.

Chacune de ces formes varie par fa longueur & par fes cavités, par fes contours extérieurs & par l'enfoncement du milieu. Chacune ne convient qu'à telle ou telle tête, chacune porte l'empreinte d'un caractère individuel.

L'oreille 1. est auffi la première en rang pour la douceur, la fimplicité, la modeftie & la candeur.

La 2de eft plus nuancée, plus fufceptible de culture.

La 3 encore plus délicate, plus fpirituelle & plus attentive que les deux précédentes.

J'ofe foutenir que la 4e ne fauroit être celle d'un homme ordinaire, mais elle eft peut-être un peu plus dure que la 3e.

La 5e eft vraifemblablement la plus originale & la plus éveillée des douze.

6. plus flegmatique que 3. 4. 5., moins fenfible que cette dernière, mais beaucoup plus capable que 1.

7. pleine d'efprit & de fineffe.

8. L'arrondiffement du contour fupérieur eft très-fingulier, je ne fais qu'en dire: feulement je doute que cette oreille ait le mérite de la précédente.

Je foupçonne la 9e d'un peu de timidité; d'ailleurs je la crois jufte & active.

La 10e me paroit infignifiante, étourdie, éventée & fade; fa facilité n'eft que brouillonnerie.

11. circonfpection dénuée de toute efpèce de courage.

12. n'admet guères les paffions violentes; j'y démêle la modeftie & la douceur, fondées fur la nobleffe du fentiment.

Planche XLIX.
                        V v

4D

Inquisition. He was reinstated only years later. Tagliacozzi's burial place is unknown at present (41, 73, 111, 112, 129, 134).

In the latter part of the same century, knowledge of surgery spread to Paris with the drive of the barber surgeons to obtain medical recognition. The most prominent and influential surgeon of his times was undoubtedly Ambroise Paré. He believed in heresy and witchcraft. Paré was miraculously saved by the king, who commanded him ro remain in the royal chambers during the fateful night of St. Bartholomew's Eve when the Huguenots were massacred. Paré condemned the Italian surgical methods. He described and illustrated a prosthesis of an ear made of enamelled metal and attached to the head by a wire hoop (Fig. 2) (41, 74, 84, 86, 111, 112, 134).

After Paré's time there was a void in ear surgery, and nothing positive was published for over 250 years. Medicine was reduced to empiricism dominated by religious symbolism. Contributions were made to anatomy of the ear in the seventeenth century by Barroco, Casserio, Du Vernay, Valsalva, Cotugno, Scarpa, Casselbohn, and others. But we can only suspect that surgery and progress were not altogether dormant. Cocherill (20) quotes an extract from Stafford (tome II, page 66) relating that during the reign of Charles I of England a common punishment for minor crimes was to nail the culprit's ears to a rack and then cut them off (1630). This happened to a minister, a lawyer, and a physician, named Burton, Prynne, and Barwick, respectively, who were condemned for having published a pamphlet that was supected of affecting the honor of the Queen. The judge was surprised to find that Prynne had been punished previously in a similar way. He was examined in court, and scars were found where his ears had been sewn back on. Prynne's ears were cut off a second time. Immediately afterward Prynne's wife ran to get them, wrapped them, and took them to a surgeon to repeat the procedure. There is no mention of the result of the second replacement. Nor is any surgeon named, who was obviously working outside the law and had to remain anonymous.

The attitude toward aesthetic ear surgery during the last century is best expressed by Chassignac (20): "These plastics are unjustified because of the danger of death, due to erisipelas." Such was the situation until asepsis changed the field. Roux (20) wrote on radical ear repair: "Where to get enough skin? or local flaps? how to form the cartilage? with the gracious curves of the concha or relief on the other side? Only a deformed similie can be hoped for. A thousand times better is a coloured artifice." "It is pretended," mentioned Troeltsch (20), "that the application of the ear of another person was practised in India with success, but no precise documents are to be had of these extraordinary things." So waned the myth, which had been repeated for two centuries, of a homograft from a "sympathetic" slave.

There were important contributions in the nineteenth century. Boyer (15) established that the treatment for microtia was amputation. Traumatic loss was more honorable than a congenital deformity, attributed at that time to hereditary syphilis. Boyer also illustrated a wedge excision for lobe repair in a child whose lobule reached down to the neck, and for tumors of the lobule. Jobert de Lamballe (61) successfully freshened the edges of a divided lobe that had been ripped by an earring. Cocherill (20) cites several case histories in England and France at the beginning of the last century with good "takes" after replacement of partial and total ear loss due to trauma. Dieffenbach (37) repaired the loss of the posterior helical border with bridge flaps from the mastoid, and similarly upward for lobule loss, in two stages, leaving the defect to heal by second intention. Dieffenbach was often cited by his contemporaries during the following decades. However, we have been unable to find precise treatment for prominent ears in his works, as it has been repeatedly published that he performed the first retroaural skin excision for this condition. The first attempt at total ear reconstruction is attributed to Szymanowski (125) who delineated the ear by rolling in skin flaps.

Old studies of beauty were elementary on the ear (Fig. 3) (104). One of the most pleas-

CHRONIQUES
VARIÉTÉS ▧ INFORMATIONS

Le portrait parlé [1]

L'OREILLE

Dans sa fable de « l'Ane vêtu de la peau du lion » le fabuliste nous montre un trompeur, démasqué sous son déguisement, par la forme de son oreille :

Un petit bout d'oreille échappé par malheur
Découvrit la fourbe et l'erreur.

Pour la reconnaissance des criminels, les policiers attachent une grande importance aux for-

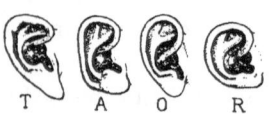

Fig. 2. — Formes générales de l'oreille.
T . triangulaire ; A : rectangulaire ; O : ovale ; R : ronde.

mes de l'oreille et considèrent la description du pavillon auriculaire comme la plus importante partie du portrait parlé.

Pour la description des diverses formes et particularités de cet organe, ils choisissent l'oreille droite ; ce n'est que dans le cas où l'oreille droite n'existe plus qu'ils décrivent l'oreille gauche. Le portrait parlé notera :

LA FORME GÉNÉRALE DE L'OREILLE est, en général, ovoïde à grosse extrémité en haut; quand elle sera caractéristique, on la cotera : triangulaire, rectangulaire, ovalaire ou ronde.

L'ÉCARTEMENT DU PAVILLON sera indiqué quand

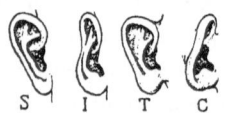

Fig. 3. — Ecartement du pavillon.
S : supérieur ; I : inférieur ; T : total ;
C : cassé à l'antitragus.

il sera notable; cet écartement peut porter sur la partie supérieure, inférieure (lobe) ou sur la

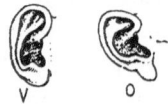

Fig. 4. — Insertion du pavillon.
V : insertion verticale ; O : insertion oblique.

totalité. L'oreille peut être collée à la tête par

1. D'après Edmond LOCARD : *Manuel de Technique policière*, 2e édition (Payot, édit.), Paris, 1934; voir *La Presse Médicale*, 16 Décembre 1936, n° 101.

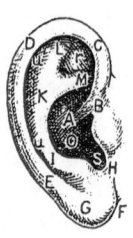

Fig. 1. — Les parties de l'oreille.
A, B : Bordure originelle. — B, C : Bordure antérieure; C, D : Bordure supérieure; D. E : Bordure postérieure; G : Lobe ; F : Point d'attache du lobe à la joue; F, H : zone d'adhérence du lobe à la joue; H, B : Tragus; H, I : antitragus; I, K : Pli inférieur; K, M : Pli médian ; O : Conque ; u, u : Fossette naviculaire ; r : Fossette digitale; S : canal antétragien.

sa bordure supérieure, ou cassée à l'antitragus (c'est-à-dire écartée du crâne, sauf dans sa partie inférieure).

L'INSERTION DU PAVILLON DE L'OREILLE. — En général, elle est un peu oblique en bas et en avant; elle sera indiquée par : verticale ou très oblique (on ne notera que les cas prononcés).

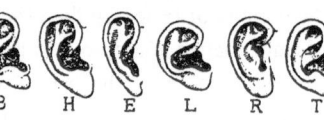

Fig. 5. — Conque.
B : basse ; H : haute ; E : étroite ; L : large ;
R : repoussée ; T : traversée.

LA CONQUE. — Au centre du pavillon auriculaire est une cavité, sorte d'antichambre du conduit auditif externe, la conque qui aboutit à ce conduit.

On ne la décrit que si elle a nettement une forme particulière : basse, haute, étroite, large; elle est dite *repoussée* quand la cavité est remplie

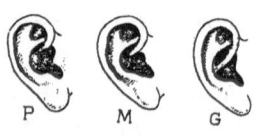

Fig. 6. — Bordure originelle.
P: petite ; M : moyenne ; G : grande.

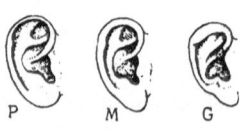

Fig. 7. — Bordure supérieure (largeur de l'ourlet).
P: petite ; M : moyenne ; G : grande.

par une saillie, *traversée* quand la bordure originelle, très longue, rejoint le pli.

On examine et on décrit ensuite successivement la BORDURE, le LOBE ou lobule, l'ANTITRAGUS, le TRAGUS, le PLI.

1° LA BORDURE. — On appelle ainsi le bourrelet qui borde les deux tiers supérieur et postérieur de l'oreille, et vient se terminer dans le lobe. On décompose la bordure, pour la description, en trois parties :

a) La *bordure originelle*, qui est le point de départ de la bordure, placée dans la conque, au creux de l'oreille ; on note sa longueur par P, M ou G (petite, moyenne ou grande).

b) La *bordure supérieure* qui est la bordure du

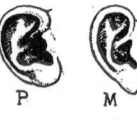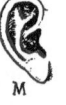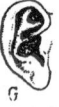

Fig. 8. — Bordure postérieure (largeur de l'ourlet).
P : petite ; M : moyenne ; G : grande.

haut de l'oreille et dont l'épaisseur se note de la même façon. (Il faut bien prendre garde que, dans la bordure originelle, c'est la longueur que l'on considère, tandis que dans les bordures supérieure et *postérieure* on ne considère que la largeur.)

On relève sur les bordures de nombreuses particularités qui sont : *a)* La *nodosité darwinienne ; b)* Le *petit point dur* à la limite des bordures supérieure et postérieure, plus facilement perceptible au toucher qu'à la vue.

c) L'*élargissement darwinien au milieu* de la

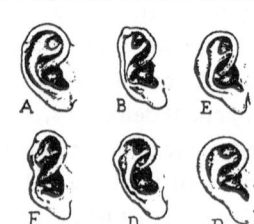

Fig. 9. — Particularités de la bordure.
A : nodosité; B : tubercule; E : élargissement;
F : bordure froissée; D : bordure échancrée;
P : bordure postérieure fondue.

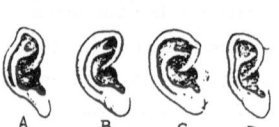

Fig. 10. — Contour du pavillon.
A : contour supérieur aigu; B : contour supérieur antérieur aigu; C : supérieur antérieur équerre; D : supérieur postérieur équerre.

A

Fig. 5A and **B.** Common malformations of the ear and their variations. From *Le Portrait Parlé*, by P. Desposses (Presse Medicale), 1937.

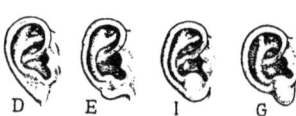

Fig. 11. — Lobe (contour).
D : descendant; E : équerre; I : intermédiaire; G : golfe.

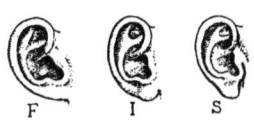

Fig. 12. — Adhérence du lobe à la joue.
F : lobe fondu; I : intermédiaire; S : lobe séparé.

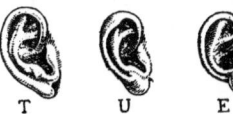

Fig. 13. — Lobe (modelé du).
T : traversé; U : uni; E : éminent.

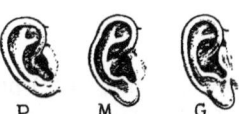

Fig. 14. — Lobe (hauteur).
P : petite; M : moyenne; G : grande.

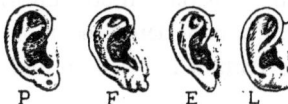

Fig. 15. — Particularités du lobe.
P : lobe percé; F : lobe fendu; E : lobe étroit; L : lobe large.

bordure postérieure ; on devra mentionner la *bordure froissée* ; la *bordure échancrée*, à l'union de la bordure supérieure et de la postérieure; la *bordure postérieure fondue* avec le pli inférieur; le *contour supérieur aigu* (oreille pointue) ; le *contour supéro-antérieur* aigu (pointe en avant), le *contour supéro-antérieur équerre*; le *contour supéro-postérieur équerre*. Ces diverses indications désignent les formes angulaires variées qui sont toutes rares; normalement le haut de l'oreille est arrondi.

2° LE LOBE. — Le lobe ou lobule termine en bas le pavillon de l'oreille ; il est constitué par une petite masse charnue, ovoïde, libre sur ses faces et adhérente à la joue, d'ordinaire seulement par la partie la plus élevée de son bord antérieur.

On note son contour, son adhérence à la joue, son modelé et sa hauteur.

a) Le contour peut se terminer en bas par une *pointe* (descendant), par une *équerre*, par une *courbe* partiellement adhérente à la joue (*intermédiaire*), par une courbe entièrement libre (*golfe*) ;

b) L'adhérence à la joue peut être sans ride ni sillon (*fondue*), incomplète (*intermédiaire*), avec un sillon plus ou moins profond (*séparée*);

c) Le modelé du lobe peut être *traversé* s'il y a un pli horizontal, ou *uni*, ou *éminent* si le lobe forme une saillie convexe ;

d) La hauteur, enfin, peut être *petite, moyenne* ou *grande* ;

e) Quant aux particularités, on relèvera le lobe *percé* (boucles d'oreilles), *fendu, étroit, large*, à *fossette*, à *virgule* (fossette longue), à *tlot* (fossette bifurquée), etc...

3° ANTITRAGUS (fig. 19). — L'antitragus est la saillie située en bas de la conque et au-dessus du lobe. On le considère au point de vue de son inclinaison, de son profil, de son renversement et de son volume.

a) L'inclinaison de l'antitragus varie entre *horizontale, intermédiaire* et *oblique* ;

b) Le profil est le degré de concavité ou de convexité de l'antitragus et se décrit par les termes : *cave, rectiligne, intermédiaire, saillant* ;

c) Le renversement de l'antitragus, en dehors de la conque, se marque par *versé, intermédiaire* et *droit* ;

d) Le volume est *petit, moyen, grand* ;

e) Les particularités sont : l'antitragus *fusionné* avec la bordure originelle au fond de la conque ; l'*incisure post-antitragienne* (ride en arrière de l'antitragus) ; le *canal étroit* (peu de distance entre l'antitragus et l'autre saillie placée en face et appelée tragus).

4° LE TRAGUS est cette saillie placée en avant de la conque et qui abrite l'entrée du conduit auditif; le tragus est un peu plus haut que l'antitragus. On note seulement les particularités : *tragus poilu, tragus bifurqué.*

5° LE PLI. — C'est la saillie courbe placée

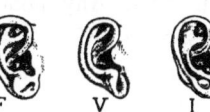

Fig. 16. — Autres particularités du lobe.
F : lobe à fossettes; V : lobe à virgule; I : lobe à tlot.

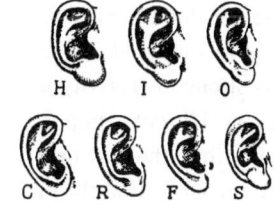

Fig. 17. — Antitragus (inclinaison et profil).
H : horizontal; I : intermédiaire; O : oblique; C : cave; R : rectiligne; F : intermédiaire; S : saillant.

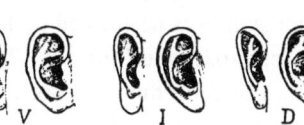

Fig. 18. — Antitragus (renversement).
V : versé; I : intermédiaire; D : droit.

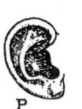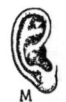

Fig. 19. — Volume de l'antitragus.
P : petit; M : moyen; G : grand.

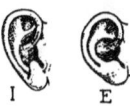

Fig. 20. — Antitragus (particularités).
I : incisure post. antitragienne; E : canal étroit.

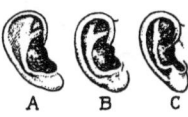

Fig. 21. — Pli supérieur.
A : effacé; B : intermédiaire; C : accentué.

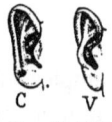

Fig. 22. — Pli inférieur.
C : cave; V : convexe.

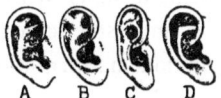

Fig. 23. — Particularités du pli.
A : pli supérieur à plusieurs branches; B : pli joignant la bordure; C : hématome; D : pli médian horizontal.

entre la conque en avant et la bordure en arrière; on la divise en pli supérieur et pli inférieur. Le pli supérieur se classe suivant son degré de saillie en *effacé, intermédiaire* ou *accentué*; le pli inférieur en *cave, intermédiaire* ou *convexe* ; pour cet examen, il faut se placer en face de l'individu et voir si le pli dépasse ou non la bordure. Le pli peut offrir les particularités suivantes : *pli supérieur à plusieurs branches, pli supérieur joignant la bordure, hématome* (petite bosse sanguine sur le pli supérieur), *pli médian horizontal.*

**

On le voit, le pavillon auriculaire, sorte de cornet aplati dont la paroi est plusieurs fois repliée sur elle-même, offre un assemblage de formes singulières qui varient beaucoup suivant les sujets ; si on note un nombre suffisant de ces formes, il est impossible de confondre une oreille avec une autre oreille; c'est ce qui donne à cet organe tant de valeur pour le portrait parlé.

P. DESFOSSES.

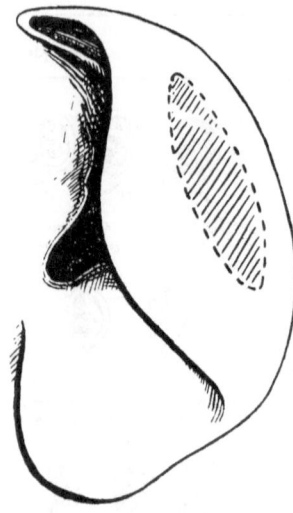

Fig. 6. Classical illustration of a true "lop" ear. From *Essai sur la restauration du pavillon de l'oreille,* by R. Cocherill, 1894.

ing examples of medical aesthetics is Lavater's "Essai sur la Physionomie," (72) published in four scholarly tomes. They cover in detail every part of the face and expression, but only 3 pages are devoted to the ear (Fig. 4). Dürer printed excellent studies of the face, but the designs of the ear were distorted. Any modern aesthetic surgeon will do well to read an aesthetic analysis by Desposses (35, 36), who carefully considered the more common malformations of the ear and their variations in "le Portrait Parlé: l'Oreille" (Fig. 5).

The first paper on record for correction of prominent ears is by Ely (1, 40). The paper is particularly eloquent because of the humility of Ely, who states that his technique may not be the first: "I do not know whether this is a new operation . . . but, if allowed to judge from a single case, I can highly recommend it." Ely was an ophthalmo-otologist who practised in New York City. His strenuous activity undermined his fragile health, and he died of tuberculosis at the age of 35. His contribution to correction of prominent ears consisted of operating on one ear at a time, the first on March 1 and the second on April 19, 1881. He incised straight through from behind the ear, including all layers, and the freer border adhered to the mastoid with healing by second intention.

Removal of an ellipse of skin and underlying cartilage from the retroaural sulcus, without cutting through the anterior skin, was performed by Keen (66), Monks and Pearl (87), Haug (20), Cocherill (20), Joseph (62), and Morestin (71, 88).

It soon became evident that this procedure did not produce a sufficient or permanent result, and several surgeons developed methods of fixation of the cartilage to the mastoid surface. Thus, Gersuny (49) sutured the perichondrium to the mastoid periosteum; Malbec

(80, 81) used "orthopaedic stitches"; Ruttin (109) anchored the cartilage with fascia lata strips; and Payr (100) and later Demel and Feigl (34) embedded a cartilage flap under the periosteum. Cartilage fixation to the mastoid has recently been revived by Paletta et al. (97), Furnas (48), Spira et al. (116), and Reichert (107). Nicoletis (93) has developed an interesting variation of mastoid fixation by disinserting the auricularis posterior muscle from the concha and reattaching it to the scapha, thus basculating the pinna.

A fundamental step came with the famous contribution of Luckett (2, 78), who established that the basic deformity of prominent ear was the flattening of the antihelix. His approach was from the posterior aspect, incising skin and excising a cresecent of underlying cartilage along the antihelical line; the cartilage edges were bent over with Lempert stitches. Luckett was born in Texas, graduated from medical school in Virginia, became chief of surgery in Harlem and Lutheran hospitals in New York City, and was a champion pistol shot in the United States. The value of his conception was rapidly understood, and the technique was repeated with minor modifications. Young (136) prolonged the cartilage incision to break the spring and avoid suturing, Barsky (7) beveled the borders, Jones (60) excised a wider cartilage strip, and Vidaurre (132) added an incision for the anterior crus. Jayes and Dale (59) and Spina (114) also used antihelical incisions.

However, it was found that all these procedures resulted in a sharp antihelical ridge instead of the normal curve. Surgeons devised a series of techniques to try to decrease the sharpness. The earliest attempts were parallel incisions of the cartilage instead of a single one [Baxter (9), Fernandez (45), Pierce et al. (102), Mc Evitt (85), Erich (42), Friedman (46), Farina et al. (43)]. These longitudinal incisions were cross-hatched by Borges (13). The cartilage was thinned on the posterior aspect with brush abrasion by Farrior (44). Patton (99) used a gouge to do the same thing after removing the perichondrium, and Holmes (58) cut oblique shingling incisions as fish scales. All were a step forward, although none was perfect.

To cover these visible cartilage ridges, some authors have kept an intact segment of cartilage over the cartilage incisions by suturing the cut edges under a bridge [Barsky (7), Becker (1o)], tubing the strip after thinning it with abrasion [Converse and Wood-Smith (21)], or rolling it like a cornucopia [Tanzer (127,128)] or an island [Pitanguy and Rebello (103)].

In his last of three cases, Morestin (88) used a different approach. Instead of treating the cartilage, he simply bent it and held it in place with nonabsorbable sutures. Luckett (78) wrote: "In an ear with a very thin flexible cartilage I think it would be possible to reconstruct the antihelix and set the helix close to the head without excising a segment, or even incising the cartilage, simply by fluting or folding the cartilage at the proper site, and passing the suture in such a manner as to maintain the fold." This method was presented by Owens and Delgado (95) but was greatly refined and popularized by Mustardé (91).

During recent years another approach has been developed. Byars (25, 27) observed that if a rib cartilage is incised, it curls toward the intact perichondrium. This was studied experimentally by Gibson and Davis (50), and especially by Stenström (118,120) in ear cartilage. Tamerin and Mirehouse (126) put this principle into practice by attacking the lateral antihelical surface with multiple partial-thickness incisions. This procedure was repeated by Paletta et al. (97) and Crikelair and Cosman (23), scored by Chongchet (17). Stark and Saunders (117) reduced the surface with a brush. The technique was further refined by Cloutier (19), who incised right through the cartilage from behind and beveled the edges so that they curled and overlapped. Reichert (107) reached the anterior surface in a similar way through a Y incision, and scored the lateral aspect. Davis (24, 26) has performed lateral surface hand abrasion of the cartilage, simultaneously with a relaxing scaphal dome incision, keeping the scapha and helix independent. All these methods undoubtedly have produced a softer curved and more natural antihelix without requiring foreign material to hold the position.

Another type of ear prominence is due to a high concha. Surgeons have used various approaches to correct this defect. The posterior wall of the concha has been incised and overlapped [Alexander (4), Young (136), Marino (83), and Aubry et al. (6)]; strips of cartilage have been removed from the concha [Kitlowski (67), Peet and Paterson (101)]; and the conchal cartilage floor has been completely removed [Davis (24, 26)].

A further approach has been to reduce the prominence with simple procedures that hardly require bandaging. These have been through skin stab wounds, and the cartilage was treated after raising the skin over the antihelical area. Thus, Gonzalez-Ulloa (52) performed full-thickness incisions of the cartilage along the antihelical line and held the position with fine wire stitches. Stenström (118,120) made multiple partial-thickness incisions on the lateral surface with a special multiple-blade instrument, and Kaye (65) did a similar thing with the teeth of a dissecting forceps.

Prominent ears are frequently associated with abnormal positions of the antitragus. Repositioning the antitragus has been performed with cross-hatching by Mc Evitt (85) or by incising the cartilage subtotally to allow it to bend, and sliding the skin over it to hold the new position [Davis (26)]. The lobule can also stand out after the scapha is reduced, and it has been set back by removing a horizontal triangle of skin [Baumgarter (8)], by suturing the tail of the helix to the concha [Goulian and Conway (55), Rubin et al. (108)], or by combining antihelical cartilage tail excision with removal of an anterior lobular wedge [Davis (25, 26)].

Correction of cryptotia, pocket, or invaginated ears was apparently first described by Kubo (70), who lowered a skin flap. The method was improved by Sercer (110), who performed a YV advancement, and later by Gosserez and Piers (53), who did a Z-plasty and graft. Cowan (22) more carefully considered the causes of this deformity.

Lop ears have been corrected by accentuation of the upper crus by cartilage excision and suture, as seen in Fig. 6 [Cocherill (20)]. The position is held by transfixion on a bolus [Eckstein (39)] or by everting stitches [Joseph (63)]. Ragnell (105) reshaped the cartilage with a zigzag expansion incision and held the new position with a wire hoop for 3 months. Grotting (57) brought a retroauricular flap forward to fill the gap after anterior helical expansion. Stephenson (121) used a fan incision of the helix, which Musgrave (90) reinforced with a helical cartilaginous bridge. Stenström (120) performed a VY composite advancement, and Davis (27, 28) fashioned an expansion by transposing a cartilage peninsula from the cymba to the fossa triangularis.

Scafoid or shell ears have been corrected by accentuating the helical curve with multiple wedge removal [Padgett and Stephenson (96)], scratching the medial surface to allow the cartilage to bend [Stenström (120)], and pulling the helix forward after a triangular excision of the helical head and removing excess scapha [Davis (25)].

Even during the last century there was considerable interest in macrotia, and one may suspect that many prominent ears were treated by reducing their size. Different designs and combinations of triangular excisions were used. The first was developed by Giuseppe Di Martino (38), and later contributions have been by Trendelenburg et al. (130), Joseph (62), Gersuny (49), Cheyne and Burghard (16), and Day (31). More recently, triangular excisions have been avoided with an effort to limit tissue removal to the scaphahelical sulcus area as a long curved strip. The independent helix is then readapted to the reduced scapha, and either the tail is removed [Ju et al. (64)] or the head is excised [Davis (24, 25)].

Aging of ears has been classified and considered essentially a lobular deformity. Treatment is by reduction or augmentation [Davis (29)], which is added in face-lifting operations by partial lobule excision [Loeb (76)].

In summary, there is a scarcity of literature on ear repair as compared with other fields in aesthetic surgery. The history of aesthetic surgery of the ear has been a delayed explosion which occurred in slightly more than a century, gaining momentum and finally booming in recent years. Different parts of the ear were corrected separately until Foman et al. (47) considered the ear as a whole, and finally Davis (24, 26) stated that the result of ear surgery should look pleasing and be normal. For a pleasant appearance the ear must be in balance with the size of the head, and the different parts of the ear must be balanced among themselves. To be normal the ear must show no sign of surgery. This integral conception of the organ, and the perfection of results, is what makes or breaks the aesthetic surgeon.

References

1. A classic reprint. An operation for prominence of the auricles. Edward T. Ely. Commentary by Blair O. Rogers. Plast. Reconst. Surg. 42:582, 1968.
2. A classic reprint. A new operation for prominent ears based on the anatomy of the deformity. William H. Luckett. Commentary by Blair O. Rogers. Plast. Reconstr. Surg. 43:83, 1969.
3. A classic reprint. Ancient ear-lobe and rhinoplastic operations in India (from the Susruta Samhita). Translated from the Sanskrit and published by K. K. L. Bhishagratna, Calcutta, 1907. Commentary by Frank McDowell. Plast. Reconstr. Surg. 43:515, 1969.
4. Alexander, G.: Zur plastischen Korrektur abstehender ohrmuscheln. Wien. Klin. Wochenschr. 41:1217, 1928.
5. Alexander, G.: Zur Technik der Plastischen Operationem am aeusseren Ohre. Z. Hals-, Nasen-, Ohrenh. 21:6, 1928.
6. Aubry, M., Jost, G., and Neveu, M.: Simplified technique for protruding ears. Procedure of Hector Marino. Ann. Otolaryngol. 79:587, 1962.
7. Barsky, A. J.: Plastic Surgery. W. B. Saunders Co., Philadelphia, 1938.

8. Baumgartner, P. H.: A technical hint for the correction of prominent ears. Based on the method of Converse. Plast. Reconstr. Surg. 37:66, 1966.

9. Baxter, H.H.: Prominent ears. Can. Med. Assoc. J. 45:217, 1941.

10. Becker, O. J.: Correction of the protruding deformed ear. Br. J. Plast. Surg. 5: 187, 1952.

11. Binnie, J. F.: Manual of Operative Surgery. Blakiston's Son and Co., Philadelphia, 1921.

12. Bhishagratna, K. K. L.: An English Translation of the Susruta Samhita. Wilkins Press, Calcutta, 1907.

13. Borges, A. F.: Prominent ears: Modification of Dr. Forrest Young's technique. Plast. Reconstr. Surg. 12:208, 1952.

14. Bourgery, J. M.: Traité Complet de l'Anatomie de l'Homme. C. A. Delaunay, Paris, 1840.

15. Boyer, M. le Baron: Traité des Maladies Chirurgicales et des Opérations qui leur Conviennent. Migneret, Paris, 1822.

16. Cheyne, W. W. and Burghard, S. F.: Manual of Surgical Treatment. Longmans, Green and Co., London, 1903.

17. Chongchet, V.: A method of antihelix reconstruction. Br. J. Plast. Surg. 16:268, 1963.

18. Cloquet, J.: Anatomie de l'Homme. C. de Lasteyrie, Paris, 1822.

19. Cloutier, A. MacLeod: Correction of outstanding ears. Plast. Reconstr. Surg. 28:412, 1961.

20. Cocherill, R.: Essai sur la restauration du pavillon de l'oreille. Thèses, Lille, 1894.

21. Converse, J. M. and Wood-Smith, D.: Technical details in the surgical correction of lop ear deformity. Plast. Reconstr. Surg. 31:118, 1963.

22. Cowan, R. J.: Cryptotia. Plast. Reconstr. Surg. 27:209, 1961.

23. Crikelair, G. F. and Cosman, B.: Another solution for the problem of the prominent ear. Ann. Surg. 160:324, 1964.

24. Davis, J. E.: On prominent ears. Transactions of the V International Congress on Plastic and Reconstructive Surgery. Butterworths, Melbourne, 1971.

25. Davis, J. E.: On auricular construction. Microf. J. Aesthet. Plast. Surg. 1972-A.

26. Davis, J. E.: Complications of prominent ear surgery. Microf. J. Aesthet. Plast. Surg. 1972-B.

27. Davis, J. E.: Auricle reconstruction. Reviews in Plastic Surgery: General Plastic and Reconstructive Surgery. Excerpta Medica, Amsterdam, 1974.

28. Davis, J. E.: Repair of severe cup ear deformities. Symposium on Reconstruction of the Auricle. C. V. Mosby Co., St. Louis, 1974.

29. Davis, J. E.: Envejecimiento de la Oreja. Segundo Congreso Argentino de Cirugía Estética. Buenos Aires, 1974.

30. Davis, J. S.: Plastic Surgery, Its Principles and Practise. P. Blakiston's Son and Co., Philadelphia, 1919.

31. Day, H. F.: Reconstruction of the ears. Boston Med. Surg. J. 185:146, 1921.

32. Davenport, G. and Bernard F. D.: Experience with mattress suture technique in correction of prominent ears. Plast. Reconstr. Surg. 36:91, 1965.

33. Dembo, A. and Imbelloni, J.: Deformidades Intencionales del Cuerpo Humano de caracter Etnico. Biblioteca del Americanista Moderno, Buenos Aires. 1947.

34. Demel, R. and Feigl, E.: The correction of prominent ears. Dtsch. Z. Chir. 233:453, 1931.

35. Desposses, P.: Le portrait parlé: l'oreille. Presse Med. 20:561, 1937.

36. Desposses, P.: Le portrait parlé. l'oreille. Presse Med. 101: 2049, 1936.

37. Dieffenbach, J. F.: Die Operative Chirurgie. F. A. Brockhaus, Leipzig, 1845.

38. Di Martino, G.: Anomalie du pavillon de l'oreille et procédé d'otomiose. Bull. Acad. Med. Paris 22:17, 1857.

39. Eckstein, E.: Ohrmuschelfaltung zur Beseitigung des Abstehens der Ohrmuschel. Verh. Dtsch. Ges. Chir. 41:84, 1912.

40. Ely, E. T.: An operation for prominent auricles. Arch. Otolaryngol. 10:97, 1881.

41. Entralgo, P. L.: Grandes Médicos. Salvat, Barcelona, 1961.

42. Erich, J. B.: Surgical correction of protruding ears. Mayo Clin. Proc. 33:99, 1958.

43. Farina, R., Baroudi, R., Coleman, B., and De Castro, O.: Otoplasty. Br. J. Plast. Surg. 15:194, 1962.

44. Farrior, R. T.: A method of otoplasty. A.M.A. Arch. Otolaryngol. 69:400, 1959.

45. Fernandez, J.: Orejas en asa. Técnica personal. Rev. Asoc. Med. Argentina 30:1019, 1943.

46. Friedman, H. S.: Otoplasty. A.M.A. Arch. Otolaryngol. 70:454, 1959.

47. Fomon, S., Bell, J. W., Lubart, J., Schnattner, A. and Syracuse, V. R.: The problem of outstanding ears. A. M. A. Arch. Otolaryngol. 71:753, 1960.

48. Furnas, D.: Correction of prominent ears by conchamastoid sutures. Plast. Reconstr. Surg. 42:189, 1968.

49. Gersuny, R.: Uber einige kosmetische Operationen. Wien. Med. Wochenschr. 53:2253, 1903.

50. Gibson, T. and Davis, W. B.: The distortion of autogenous cartilage grafts: Its cause and prevention. Brt. J. Plast. Surg. 10:257, 1958.

51. Goldstein, Operative Surgery of the Nose, Throat and Ear (Lobe). C. V. Mosby Co., St. Louis, 1917.

52. Gonzalez-Ulloa, M.: An easy method to correct prominent ears. Br. J. Plast. Surg. 4:207, 1951.

53. Gosserez, M. and Piers, J. H.: Invagination congenital du pavillon de l'oreille. Ann. Chir. Plast. 4:143, 1959.

54. Gottlieb, F. M.: Die Behandlung abstehender Ohren. Thesis, Berlin, 1932.

55. Goulian, D. and Conway, H.: Prevention of persistent deformity of the tragus and lobule by modification of Luckett's technique of otoplasty. Plast. Reconstr. Surg. 26:399, 1960.

56. Graham, H. B.: Plastic surgery of the ear. West J. Surg. 44:478, 1936.

57. Grotting, J. K.: Otoplasty for congenital cupped protruding ears using a postauricular flap. Plast. Reconstr. Surg. 22:164, 1958.

58. Holmes, E. M.: A new procedure for correcting outstanding ears. A.M.A. Arch. Otolaryngol. 69:409, 1959.

59. Jayes, P. H. and Dale, R. H.: The treatment of prominent ears. Br. J. Plast. Surg. 4:193, 1951.

60. Jones, E. H.: Operation for the correction of protruding ears. South. Med. J. 52:1067, 1959.

61. Jobert, A. J. (de Lamballe): Traité de Chirurgie Plastique. J. B. Baillière, Paris, 1849.

62. Joseph, J.: Report of a lecture at meeting of October 21, 1896. Verh. Berl. Med. Ges. 27:206, 1896.

63. Joseph, J.: Korrektive Nasen und Ohrenplastik. Handbuch der Speziellen Chirurgie des Ohres. Katz & Blumfeld, Leipzig, 1921.

64. Ju, D. M. C., Li, C. and Crikelair, G. F.: The surgical correction of protruding ears. Plast. Reconstr. Surg. 32:283, 1963.

65. Kaye, B. L.: Simplified method of correcting prominent ear. Plast. Reconstr. Surg. 40:44, 1967.

66. Keen, W. W.: A new method of operating for relief of deformity of prominent ears. Ann. Surg. 11:40, 1890.

67. Kitlowski, E. A.: Correction of prominent ears. Plast. Reconstr. Surg. 23:375, 1959.

68. Kolle, F. S.: Plastic and Cosmetic Surgery. D. Appleton & Co., New York, 1911.

69. Kristensen, H. K.: Correction of outstanding ears. Ugeskr. Laeger 114:517, 1952.

70. Kubo, I.: Uber das "Taschenohr" (Kubo) und die plastische Operation dieser Missbildung. Otologia 6:105, 1933.

71. Lalardrie, J. P.: Hippolyte Morestin (1869–1981). Br. J. Plast. Surg. 25:39, 1972.

72. Lavater, J. G.: Essai sur la Physionomie (Vol. III). Jaques Van Karnebeek, La Haye, 1783.

73. Lernoud, P.: Historia de la Otología. Clínica y Cirugía Otológica. Bibliográfica Argentina, Buenos Aires. 1958.

74. Les Oeuvres d'Ambroise Paré. Pierre Rigaud, Lyon. 1652.

75. Loeb, H. W.: Operative Surgery of the Nose, Throat and Ear. C. V. Mosby Co., St. Louis, 1917.

76. Loeb, R.: Correçao da hipertrofia do lobulo auricular. Rev. Lat.-Am. Cir. Plast. 9:186, 1965.

77. Lombroso, C.: L'Homme Criminel. Baillière et Cie, Paris, 1887.

78. Luckett, W. H.: A new operation for prominent ears based on the anatomical deformity. Surg. Genecol. Obstet. 10:635, 1910.

79. Luthi, A.: Eine einfache zuverlaessige gut dosierbare Methode zur Korrektur abstehender Ohren. Schweiz. Med. Wochenschr. 10:1268, 1929.

80. Malbec, E.: Casos de cirugía estética. Rev. Cir. Med. Argentina I: 221, 1926.

81. Malbec, E.: Casos de cirugía estética. Rev. Cir. Med. Argentina Centro Est. March, 1927.

82. Maisels, D. O.: External ear anomalies. Reviews in Plastic Surgery. Excerpta Medica, Amsterdam, 1974.

83. Marino, H.: Tratamiento de las Orejas en Asa. Un detalle tecnico. Bol. Trab. Soc. Cirur. Buenos Aires 13:335, 1962.

84. Masson, G. and Asselin, P.: Dictionaire Encyclopédique de Sciences Médicales. Paris, 1882.

85. McEvitt, W. G.: The problem of the protruding ear. Plast. Reconstr. Surg. 2:481, 1947.

86. Mettler, C.: History of Medicine. Blakiston Co., Philadelphia, 1947.

87. Monks, G. H.: Operations for correcting the deformity due to prominent ears. Boston Med. Surg. J. 124:84, 1891.

88. Morestin, H.: De la reposition et du plissement cosmétiques du pavillon de l'oreille. Rev. Orthop. 4:289, 1903.

89. Morse, W.: Chinese Medicine. E. B. Krumbliaat. New York, 1934.

90. Musgrave, R. H.: A variation on the correction of congenital lop ear. Plast. Reconstr. Surg. 37:394, 1966.

91. Mustardé, J. C.: The correction of prominent ears by using simple mattress sutures. Br. J. Plast. Surg. 16:170, 1963.

92. New, G. B. and Erich, J. B.: Protruding ears; a method of plastic correction. Am. J. Surg. 48:385, 1940.

93. Nicoletis, C.: Oreilles Décollées (in print). 1975.

94. Nordzell, B.: A new method for correction of prominent ears. Acta Chir. Scand. 129:316, 1965.

95. Owens, N. and Delgado, D. D.: The management of outstanding ears. South. Med. J. 58:32, 1955.

96. Padgett, E. C. and Stephenson, K. L.: Plastic and Reconstructive Surgery. Charles C. Thomas, Springfield, Ill., 1949.

97. Paletta, F., Ship, A., and Van Norman, R.: Double spring release in otoplasty for prominent ears. Am. J. Surg. 106:566, 1963.
98. Parkhill, C.: Quoted by Kolle. In: Plastic and Cosmetic Surgery. D. Appleton and Co., New York and London, 1911.
99. Patton, H. S. The use of a mastoid gouge as a tool to simplify bilateral otoplasty. Plast. Reconstr. Surg. 29:702, 1962.
100. Payr, E.: Plastische Operationen an den Ohren (Stellungsverbesserung, Verkleinerung). Arch. Klin. Chir. 78:918, 1906.
101. Peet, E. W. and Patterson, T. J. S.: The Essentials of Plastic Surgery. Blackwell, Oxford, 1963.
102. Pierce, G. W., Klabunde, E. H. and Bergeron, V. L.: Useful procedures in plastic surgery. Plast. Reconstr. Surg. 2:358, 1947.
103. Pitanguy, I. and Rebello, C.: Ansiform ears. Correction by "island" technique. Acta Chir. Plast. 4:267, 1962.
104. Porta, Giambattista della: Della Fisionomia dell' Huomo. 1623.
105. Ragnell, A.: A new method of shaping deformed ears. Br. J. Plast. Surg. 4:202, 1951.
106. Reginato, L. E.: Corección de la hipertrofia del lóbulo de la oreja. Rev.Lat. Am. Cir. Plast. 8(4):1964.
107. Reichert, H.: Correction of protruding ears by making use of the natural elasticity of the cartilage. Transactions of the V International Congress of Plastic and Reconstructive Surgeons. Butterworths, Sydney, 1971.
108. Rubin, L. R., Bromberg, B. E., Walden, R. H., and Adams, A.: An anatomic approach to the unobtrusive ear. Plast. Reconstr. Surg. 29:360, 1962.
109. Ruttin, E.: Eine Methode zur Korrektur abstehender Ohren und zum Verschluss retroaurikulärer Offnungen. Monatsschr. Ohrenh. 44:196, 1910.
110. Sercer, A.: Beitrag zur Kenntnis der Formanomalien des äusseren Ohres. Acta Otolaryngol. 20:59, 1934.
111. Sigerist, H.: A History of Medicine. University Press, Oxford, 1962.
112. Singer, C.: A Short History of Medicine. Clarendon Press, Oxford, 1962.
113. Spadafora, A. and Muñoz, B. F.: Orejas en asa. Técnica quirúrica y resultados. Prensa Med. Argentina 46:1905, 1956.
114. Spina, V.: Protruding ears. Rev. Lat. Am. Cir. Plast. 7:, 1956.
115. Spina, V. and Ludovici, O.: Prominent ears. Plast. Reconstr. Surg. 26:405, 1960.
116. Spira, M., McCrea, R., Gerow, F., and Hardy, S.: Correction of the principle deformities causing protruding ears. Plast. Reconstr. Surg. 44:150, 1969.
117. Stark, R. B. and Saunders, D. E.: Natural appearance restored to the unduly prominent ear. Br. J. Plast. Surg. 15:385, 1962.
118. Stenström, S. J.: A "natural" technique for correction of congenitally prominent ears. Plast. Reconstr. Surg. 32:509, 1963.
119. Stenström, S. J. and Bergman, F. O.: Curling tendency of various types of distortionable cartilages. Transactions of the V International Congress of Plastic and Reconstructive Surgeons. Butterworths, Sydney, 1971.
120. Stenström, S. J.: Cosmetic deformities of the ears. In: Plastic Surgery. Little, Brown and Co., Boston, 1968.
121. Stephenson, K. L.: Correction of a lop ear type deformity. Plast. Reconstr. Surg. 26:540, 1960.

122. Straith, R. E.: Antihelix reconstruction in protruding ear operation. Plast. Reconstr. Surg. 12:454, 1953.

123. Stralgo, P. L : Historia de la Medicina Moderna y Contemporánea. Cientifica Medica, Barcelona, 1963.

124. Strombeck, J. O.: Results of surgery for protruding ears. Acta Chir. Scand. 122:138, 1961.

125. Szymanowski, J. Von: Handbuch der Operativen Chirurgie. F. Vieweg und Sohn, Braunschweig, 1870.

126. Tamerin, J. A. and Mirehouse, O.: Reconstruction of the antihelix and scapha in selected cases of protruding ears. A.M.A. Arch. Otolaryngol. 70:597, 1959.

127. Tanzer, R. C.: The correction of prominent ears. Plast. Reconstr. Surg. 30:236, 1962.

128. Tanzer, R. C.: The congenital deformities of the auricle. Reconstructive Plastic Surgery. W. B. Saunders, Philadelphia, 1964.

129. Tagliacozzi, G.: De Curtorum Chirurgia per Insitionen Libri Duo. Bindonus, Venice, 1597.

130. Trendelenburg, F., Eigenbrodt, K., and Heineke, H.: Verletzungen und chirurgische Krankheiten des Gesichts. Dtsch. Chir. 33, I and II, 1886.

131. Tucker, A. L.: Promauris. Plast. Reconstr. Surg. 15:398, 1962.

132. Vidaurre, S.: Protruding ears, another method of treatment. Plast. Reconstr. Surg. 10:39, 1952.

133. Webster, G.: Cosmetic otoplasty for protrusion. Jap. J. Plast. Surg. 5:55, 1962.

134. Webster, J. P. and Gnudi, M. T.: The life and times of Gaspare Tagliacozzi. H. Reichner, Bologna, Italy, 1924.

135. Wodak, E.: The cosmetic treatment of nose and ear. Med. Klin. 20:1052, 1924.

136. Young, F.: Correction of abnormally prominent ears. Surg. Gynecol. Obstet. 77:541, 1944.

Aesthetic Plastic Surgery 2:167–176, 1978

History of Mammaplasty

J. P. Lalardrie M.D. and **R. Mouly** M.D.

Paris, France

There is no better beginning to the saga of mammaplasties than "Once Upon a Time," as the history is truly a tale of wonder that it is our pleasure to unfold.

At its source lies woman's eternal dream—beautiful, firm, and harmoniously proportioned breasts—a dream that has inspired painting, sculpture, and literature since the dawn of mankind.

The first attempts at breast surgery were purely functional and aimed primarily at relieving women of the excessive weight of their breasts, but it was not long before aesthetic considerations came to guide the hand of the surgeon.

Our story goes back no further than the close of the nineteenth century, for neither Durston in 1669 (66) nor Velpeau in 1857 (67), the first names in the literature, had plastic considerations in mind when reducing mammary volume.

In evoking the history of plastic surgery, there is a strong temptation to enumerate names and dates and to delve into the past in an attempt to discover a pioneer because originators of new ideas are often cast in the role of heroes. But it is by no means easy to determine who was responsible for a discovery and who, by cleverly exploiting it, managed to cover himself in undeserved glory. Thus in trying to separate the wheat from the chaff, the enduring from the ephemeral, we shall cite few names and focus our attention on the development of surgical principles and techniques.

The history of reduction mammaplasty

The history of reduction mammaplasty may be conveniently broken down into three phases: pre-1930, 1930–1960, and post-1960.

Pre-1930

Glandular reduction
The first step was to use the submammary surgical route described by Gaillard-Thomas in 1882 (66) for the resection of a glandular disc from the posterior part of the mammary gland.

Address reprint requests to J. P. Lalardrie, M.D., 11, Rue de la Santé, Paris 75013, France.

0364-216X/78/0002-0167 $02.00
© 1978 Springer-Verlag New York Inc.

135

This technique was used by Morestin and Guinard (46) and refined by the Swiss surgeon De Quervain (58) who in 1925, well in advance of his time, carried out a subtotal mammectomy, leaving only a small retroareolar glandular stump.

Other resection sites were suggested by a number of surgeons, including Pousson (57), Dehner, Kuster, and Verchere (66).

Glandular reduction with nipple transposition
The need soon arose to combine glandular reduction with a transposition of the areola and nipple in order to impart a pleasing form to the reduced breast.

Reduction with transplantation. An excellent solution was found by combining reduction with free transplantation of the nipple, a technique reported by Thorek in 1922 (66) and Lexer in 1925 (34). With only minor modifications and improvements, it is the only technique of this period to have survived to our day, and it still remains the solution to some extreme cases.

Reduction with transposition. But soon surgeons were attempting to combine reduction with nipple transposition. The first reduction mammaplasty worthy of the name was performed by Aubert (3) in Marseille and described by him in 1923. It was a milestone in the history of mammaplasty.

The site and the volume of the glandular resection could be varied, but nipple transposition called for more or less extensive undermining between skin and gland.

Failures of glandular reductions in the region of the nipple were soon to draw attention to the importance of taking due account of vascularization.

Both in extent and in form, glandular exereses had to maintain one or two glandular arterial pedicles for vascularization: the stump of the remaining gland had to be vascularized by either the external pedicle or the internal pedicle or both. The number and variety of the techniques suggested may well be imagined; in every case the overriding concern was to ensure a sufficient blood supply to the residual glandular stump and hence to preserve the integrity and vitality of the nipple.

Glandular reduction, nipple transposition, and glandular remodeling
Although these glandular exereses reduced the volume of the gland, its form suffered. The vascular conditions outlined above were met, but the need was to reconstruct a harmoniously proportioned glandular stump in the form of a smaller mammary gland. Hence the necessity for *glandular remodeling* after most of these resections. This represented a major step forward allowing surgery for ptosis with associated hypertrophy and paving the way for surgical treatment of ptosis as such.

Two names are linked with this advance—Biesenberger (8–10) and Schwarzmann (63). These men may be said to have achieved the real breakthrough in mammary reduction surgery.

Biesenberger resected the outer glandular segment of the breast by a long S-shaped incision going from the upper to the lower pole of the gland: he performed a glandular modeling in such a way that the lower convex and upper concave parts of the glandular section were brought together.

Schwarzmann, 3 years later, performed a similar glandular resection incorporating a periareolar desepithelialization which has since borne his name. This began a new phase in mammary plastic surgery, perhaps the most significant to date, as the vascular security of the nipple afforded by this technique in resections of the Biesenberger type with undermining between skin and gland would enable many practitioners to increase the volume of glandular resections.

1930–1960

Mammaplasty with skin-gland undermining
The outstanding names of Gillies and McIndoe (20, 37) who, just before the outbreak of World War II, perfected Biesenberger's technique, adapting it to both hypertrophy and mammary ptosis.

It is impossible to cite all the modifications proposed. They are legion. Like those of Ragnell (59) and Aufricht (4), they were all designed to allow larger exereses or a more effective remodeling of the gland (periwinkle shell, plicature etc.).

It gradually became apparent that the royal road of progress had come up against a brick wall, as this type of operation failed to take into account the basic fact of cutaneoglandular unity and more especially vascular unity, since the breast is a cutaneous gland. Leaving the nipple on a well-vascularized glandular segment offered less opportunity for exeresis: there was a limit to glandular resection beyond which it was impossible to go without risk of necrosis. To go further a new approach was called for.

After 1960

The great merit of Arie (1) was to realize as early as 1957 that it was preferable to avoid any undermining between skin and gland. The surgery of reduction mammaplasty received a new impetus as a result of operations which offered both remarkable glandular security and extensive vascular exereses.

In 1961 Pitanguy (56) performed a "keel"-shaped resection followed by suturing of the glandular surfaces. Strombeck (65) had in 1960 performed an "hourglass"-shaped resection consisting of a cylindrical anteroposterior resection of the upper part of the gland. This technique exploits the possibilities of gland exeresis to the maximum, leaving merely a sort of glandular "basket handle" which maintains the double external and internal vascularization.

Skoog (64) in 1963 carried out a very extensive inferoposterior resection with no undermining between skin and gland, creating a "nipple-bearing" dermal flap. This technique forms the basis of present developments in mammaplasties.

As early as 1943 May's (43) maneuver had foreshadowed this technique. May had already become aware of the part played by the dermal vessels in the vascularization of the nipple and had suggested retaining a cutaneous flap for vascularization which was folded back on itself for the transposition of the nipple. Believing, however, that the primary blood supply links were between nipple and gland and that the subdermal vascularization was secondary, he resected the flap, which was temporarily clamped, once the nipple's vitality seemed assured.

Many were to follow in Skoog's footsteps—Weiner et al. (69) among others.

In 1972 McKissock (37) described a technique using a vertical bipedicular dermoglandular flap, the vascularization of the nipple being provided by the perforating arteries reaching the flap via its lower part. This part is not separated from the pectoral muscle, while its upper part, essentially dermal, is folded back on itself allowing the nipple to be raised without difficulty.

Thus, by the early 1970s, particularly after the work of Skoog and Beare (6), proof had been given of the importance of subdermal vascularization allowing subtotal mammectomies and cutaneous remodeling by desepithelialization (31). A number of techniques appeared combining differing degrees of periareolar desepithelialization and subtotal mammectomy [Garcia-Padron (50), Hinderer (28), Lalardrie (31), Schrudde (62), etc.].

Some of the techniques developed in the 1960s were subsequently modified along these lines.

Thus the limit to what could be resected was no longer what was technically feasible but rather what was necessary to obtain, the ideal residual volume.

Surgical problems

We now turn to two problems which have exercised the ingenuity of surgeons throughout the history of reduction mammaplasty: breast suspension and scars.

Breast suspension
Since the earliest days surgeons have strived to find a "trick" to stabilize reduction.

Thus Pousson (57) in 1897 and Dehner in 1908 (66) attached the upper pole of the gland to the pectoralis major or to the periosteum of the third rib.

In 1927 Göbell (24) fixed the gland to the third rib by a strip of fascia lata.

The work of Biesenberger (8), Gillies, Marino (42), and McIndoe (37) on the suspension effect of glandular remodeling seemed to hold promise and was developed by Dufourmentel and Mouly (17).

Finally came the era of *dermopexies* which could be:
dermoglandular as proposed by Tessier (54),
dermomuscular as demonstrated by Hinderer (29),
dermohypodermal following Gillies and Marino (21),
dermodermal, now the most commonly employed of modern techniques and advocated by Goulian (27) in 1971 as the sole surgical means for correcting ptosis.

Scars
Once mammary plastic surgery had come of age, surgeons sought to find means of reducing the length of scars and of making them less visible.

We may single out:
Scars resulting from a single cutaneous pleat:
Horizontal—submammary in the case of Passot (52) or higher
External horizontal [Gläsmer (23)]
Vertical [Arie (1) and Mir y Mir (44)]

Scars resulting from a double pleat:
Lower
Anchor-shaped, by far the most frequent, following Gillies, McIndoe (20), Pitanguy (56), Strombeck (65), Skoog (64), etc.
Inverted T [Biesenberger; (8)] or inverted T with short internal arm [Lalardrie (32)]
Lateral

Following Holländer (30) and Marc (40), Dufourmentel and Mouly (16) have stressed the importance of a lateralized scar.

Elements of the two types have been combined, giving an L- or J-shaped scar in techniques proposed by Elbaz and Verheecke (19), Dufourmentel and Mouly (18), and Regnault (61).

Despite the efforts of all these surgeons, the price paid in terms of scarring remains a real problem and may be considered as the ultimate stumbling block in reduction mammaplasty.

The history of augmentation mammaplasty

The operative technique of augmentation mammaplasty is more straightforward since the problem is a simpler one: it involves no more than creating a greater mammary volume as we exclude from our discussion the whole area of mammary reconstruction.

Discounting Neuber in 1893 (68), it is Czerny (15) from Heidelberg in 1895 who performed the first augmentation mammaplasty. To replace the loss of substance caused by ablation of a breast adenoma, Czerny successfully transplanted a lipoma from the patient's back.

After the work of Lexer (68) in 1925 and Passot (52) in 1930, fat transplantation became commonplace, the fatty tissue being taken from the abdomen or buttocks.

In view of the high degree of resorption noted, Berson (7) in 1944 proposed using dermal-fat transplants which Peer (55) recommended to be of the largest possible volume.

The latter proved experimentally that dermal-fat transplants accompanied by fascia revascularized more rapidly. This was the heyday of dermal-fat fascia grafts used by May (43), Watson (68), Bames (5), Conway and Dietz (12), Luque (36), Winkler (70), and others.

Enthusiasm gradually waned and the epiploic free transplants proposed by Passot (53) did not succeed in making good this deficiency.

To remedy the shortcomings of these techniques, investigators proposed *local flaps*. These were either fat in the manner of Glasner (22) or Morel-Fatio and Lalardrie (45), or dermal fat derived from Maliniac's technique (39) and advocated by Marino (41) and Longacre (35) *inter alia*.

Many attempts met with failure; others were *inclusion* of preserved human skin and *injection* of paraffin practiced as early as 1899 by Gersony (66). Vegetable oils, lanolin and beeswax, and especially liquid silicones were injected following Uchida in 1961 and Conway in 1963 (13). *Prosthetic inclusions* have since earliest times constituted the easiest solution.

The first attempts appear to have been made with balls of ivory.

In 1930 Schwarzmann (66) suggested the use of glass balls, and this solution seems to have prevailed for some years for in 1942 Thorek (66) was still advocating it "in certain cases."

Plastic inclusions

Plastics made their appearance toward the end of World War II and surgeons soon came to envisage them as a solution to their problems. Levine and Hurst seem to have been the first to use them in mammary surgery.

After this time a large number of products appeared on the market, but their use in medicine was not always without problems.

We shall mention only the five products whose names have gone down in the history of mammary inclusions.

Ivalon
Ivalon (a derivative of polyvinylic alcohol) was discovered in 1949 and is spongy in texture. This product will always be associated with the name of Pangman and Wallace (51), who in 1954 performed 400 mammary implants.

Polistan
Polistan (a derivative of polyethylene) was discovered in 1950 and is also spongy with the consistency of straw (49).

We cannot mention every name associated with this product as this would amount to a rollcall of all the plastic surgeons working in the 1950s. Gonzalez-Ulloa (26) does, however, deserve special mention as he had the idea of using heat to render the surface of the inclusion smooth, so preventing a penetration of fibrous tissue: he thus attempted to transform an open-cell inclusion into one having closed-cell properties.

Etheron
Etheron (a derivative of polymethane), discovered in 1960, takes the form of a fine-textured sponge. This may explain why this type of inclusion leads to a less marked reaction of the periprosthetic tissue. Regnault (60) made an intensive study of this product.

Hydron
Hydron (a derivative of polyglycomethacrylate) was discovered in 1961. Also of spongy texture, this product seems to have enjoyed little success.

Silicones
Silicon rubbers were used for industrial purposes as early as 1945 (11) but were not used in medicine until the early fifties.

In 1953 Brown suggested using this product as a subcutaneous inclusion.

Between 1960 and 1962 Cronin and Gerow developed a mammary silastic prosthesis, and this was first used by Gerow in March 1962 (11).

At the Third International Congress for Plastic and Reconstructive Surgery in Washington in 1963 (14), they proved that the so-called closed silastic prostheses (as against the open prostheses referred to above) brought about only a slight fibrous reaction in the surrounding area. In order to give the breast a "natural feel to the touch," Cronin and Gerow, comparing the breast to a plastic bag filled with liquid, conceived a prosthesis formed by a silastic envelope containing a gel of the same product.

From 1964 on, this type of prosthesis was used by most surgeons, and a host of publications testified to the excellent results it afforded.

At the same time Akiyama, working in Japan as early as 1949 (48), produced prostheses with an organosilicone base, having identical properties.

In 1965 Arion (2) in France created a "silicone elastomer" prosthesis which could be inflated.

The satisfactory tolerance of medical silicones over 15 years has led to the appearance of various types of prostheses. It would be impossible to list all of them, particularly as new ones are appearing all the time.

It is possible, for example, to vary the shape, contents, outer covering, and other features to meet what are often contradictory needs.

We should also mention the site of the inclusion and the route by which it is introduced. But perhaps it is well to stop here for the story is by no means over and the time has not yet come to write a complete history.

Conclusion

This, then, is the history of mammaplasty; no doubt more remains to be said and our presentation is necessarily subjective. The tale is nonetheless a fascinating one as it testifies to the work of plastic surgeons for more than a century. The best way of bringing it to life is to perform a mammaplasty. Let us be aware that each of our acts, in its ease and simplicty, bears witness to this history and to the endeavours of the men who made it.

References

1. Arie, G.: Una nueva tecnica de mastoplastia. Rev. Lat. Am. Cir. Plast. 3:23–38, 1957.
2. Arion, H. G.: Prothèses rètro-mammaires. C.R. Soc. Fr. Gynecol. 35:427–321, 1965.
3. Aubert, V.: Hypertrophie mammaire de la puberté.
4. Aufricht, J.: Mammaplasty for pendulous breast. Empiric and geometric planning. Plast. Reconstr. Surg. 4:13–29, 1949.
5. Bames, H. O.: Augmentation mammaplasty by lipi-transplant. Plast. Reconstr. Surg. 11:404–412, 1953.
6. Beare, R.: Reduction mammaplasty. Oral presentation at the Fourth International Congress for Plastic and Reconstructive Surgery, Rome, October 1967.

7. Berson, M.: Dermo-fat transplants used in building up the breast. Surgery 15:451–456, 1945.

8. Biesenberger, H.: Eine neue Methode der Mammaplastik. Zentralbl. Chir. 38:2382–2387, 1928.

9. Biesenberger, H.: Eine neue Methode der Mammaplastik. Zentralbl. Chir. 48:2971–2975, 1930.

10. Biesenberger, H.: Blutversorgung und zirkulare Umschneidung des Warzenhofes. Zentralbl. Chir. 62:1218–1223, 1935.

11. Braley, S. A.: The use of silicone in plastic surgery. A retrospective view. *Plast. Reconstr. Surg.* 51:280–288, 1973.

12. Conway, H., and Dietz, G. H.: Augmentation mammaplasty. Surg. Gynecol. Obstet. 114:573–579, 1962.

13. Cronin, T. D.: Some variations in technic in the use of silastic gel breast prothesis. First Congress of the International Society of Aesthetic Plastic Surgery, Rio de Janeiro, Feb. 6–11, 1972.

14. Cronin, T. D., and Gerow, F. J.: Augmentation mammaplasty: a new "natural feel" prothesis. Transactions of the Third International Congress of Plastic and Reconstructive Surgery, Washington, 1963. Excerpta Medica, Amsterdam, 1963, pp. 41–49.

15. Czerny, V.: Plastischer Ersatz der Brustdrüse durch ein Lipom. Zentralbl. Chir. 27:72, 1895.

16. Dufourmentel, C., and Mouly, R.: Plastie mammaire par la méthode oblique. Ann. Chir. Plast. 6:45–58, 1961.

17. Dufourmentel, C., and Mouly, R.: Modification of "periwinkleshell operation" for small ptotic breast. Plast. Reconstr. Surg. 41:523–527, 1968.

18. Dufourmentel, C., and Mouly, R.: Evolution de la méthode oblique latérale de plastie mammaire pour hypertrophie et ptose. In: J. P. Lalardrie and J. P. Jouglard (eds.): Chirurgie Plastique du Sein. Masson, Paris, 1974, pp. 106–114.

19. Elbaz, J. S., and Verheecke, G.: La cicatrice en L dans les plasties mammaires. Ann. Chir. Plast. 17:283–292, 1972.

20. Gillies, H., and McIndoe, A. H.: The technique of mammaplasty in conditions of hypertrophy of the breast. Surg. Gynecol. Obstet. 68:658–665, 1939.

21. Gillies, H., and Marino, H.: L'opération en colimaçon ou rotation spirale dans les ptôses mammaires modérées. Ann. Chir. Plast. 3:89–90, 1958.

22. Glaesmer, E.: Die Formfehler und die plastischen Operationen der weiblichen Brust. Ferd. Enke, Stuttgart, 1930.

23. Glaesmer-Zaeff, M.: Uber Mammaplastik. Zentralbl. Gynaekol., 72:1106–1116, 1950.

24. Göbell: Über autoplastische freie Fascien—und Aponeurosentransplantation nach Martin Kirchner. Arch. Klin. Chir. 146:478–480, 1927.

25. Goldwyn, R. M.: Plastic and Reconstructive Surgery of the Breast. Boston, Little, Brown and Co., 1976.

26. Gonzalez-Ulloa, M.: Correction of hypotrophy of the breast by means of exogenous material. Plast. Reconstr. Surg. 25:15–26, 1960.

27. Goulian, D., Jr.: Dermal mastopexy. Plast. Reconstr. Surg. 43:478–480, 1969.

28. Hinderer, U.: Primera experiencia con una nueva technica de mastoplastia para ptosis ligeras. Not. Med. 6:26, 1969.

29. Hinderer, U.: Remodelling mammaplasty with superficial and retromammary dermo-

pexy. 1st. Cong. I.S.A.P.S., 1972, Rio de Janeiro. Int. Microform. J. Aesth. Plast. Surg., 1972.

30. Holländer, E.: Die kosmetische Chirurgie. Vexit and Co., Leipzig, 1922, pp. 708–710.

31. Lalardrie, J. P.: The "dermal vault" technique. Reduction mammaplasty for hypertrophy with ptosis. Transacta der III Tagung der Vereinigung der Deutschen plastischen Chirurgen. Köln, 1972, pp. 105–108.

32. Lalardrie, J. P., and Jouglard, J. P.: Chirurgie Plastique du Sein. Masson, Paris, 1974.

33. Lalardrie, J. P., and Morel-Fatio, D.: Mammectomie totale sous-cutanée suivie de reconstruction immédiate ou secondaire. Mém. Acad. Chir. 96:651–662, 1970.

34. Lexer, E.: Zur Operation der Mammahypertrophie und der Hängebrust. Dtsch. Med. Wochenschr. 51:26, 1925.

35. Longacre, J. J.: The use of local pedicle flaps for reconstruction of the breast after subtotal or total extirpation of the mammary gland and for the correction of distortion and atrophy of the breast due to excessive scar. Plast. Reconstr. Surg. 11:380–403, 1953.

36. Luque, D. F.: Aumento de mamas con injertos dermo-grasos. Ann. Acad. Med-Quir. Esp. 79:225–230, 1962.

37. McIndoe, A. H.: Review of 80 cases of mammaplasty. Rev. Chir. Structive 8:39–47, 1938.

38. McKissock, P. K.: Reduction mammaplasty with a vertical dermal flap. Plast. Reconstr. Surg. 49:245–252, 1972.

39. Maliniac, J. W.: Breast Deformities and Their Repair. Grune & Stratton, New York, 1950.

40. Marc, H.: La Plastie Mammaire par la "Méthode Oblique." G. Doin, Paris, 1952.

41. Marino, E.: Extirpación total de la glandula mammaria. Reconstrucción immediata con un colgajo dermo-graso bipediculado. Prensa Med. Argent. 50:1427–1433, 1963.

42. Marino, H.: A review of new trends in corrective mammaplasty. Transactions of the Third International Congress of Plastic Surgery, Washington, Oct. 1963. Excerpta Medica, Amsterdam, 1964, pp. 66–73.

43. May, H.: Reconstruction of breast deformities. Surg. Gynecol. Obstet. 77:523–529, 1943.

44. Mir y Mir, L.: Reduction mammaplasty. Plast. Reconstr. Surg. 41:352–355, 1968.

45. Morel-Fatio, D., and Lalardrie, J. P.: Plastie mammaire d'augmentation. Ann. Chir. Plast. 11:247–250, 1966.

46. Morestin, H., and Guinard, A.: Hypertrophie mammaire traitée par la résection discoïde. Bull. Soc. Chir. (Paris) 33:649–651, 1907.

47. Murray, D. S.: Breast augmentation with gluteal dermo-fat grafts: a 5–10 year follow-up. Brt. J. Plast. Surg. 24:1–4, 1976.

48. Mutou, Y.: Augmentation mammaplasty with the Akiyama prosthesis. Brt. J. Plast. Surg. 23:58–62, 1970.

49. Neuman, Z.: The use of the non-absorbable polyethylene sponge "polystan sponge" as a subcutaneous prothesis. Brt. J. Plast. Surg. 9:195–199, 1957.

50. Padron, J. G.: Mammareduktionsplastik. Transacta der III Tagung der Vereinigung der Deutschen plastischen Chirurgen, Köln, 1972, pp. 85–87.

51. Pangman, W. J., and Wallace, R. M.: The use of plastic prothesis in breast plastic and other soft tissue surgery. West. J. Surg. 65:503–512, 1955.

52. Passot, R.: La Chirurgie Esthétique Pure. Doin, Paris, 1931, pp. 222–259.

53. Passot, R.: Atrophie mammaire: réfection esthétique par la greffe graisseuse épiploïque. Presse Méd. 37:627–629, 1930.

54. Pastoriza, J.: Hypertrophie et ptôse mammaires. Gaz. Méd. Fr. 75:5569–5593, 1968.

55. Peer, R. A.: A loss of weight and volume in human fat grafts. Plast. Reconstr. Surg. 5:217–230, 1950.

56. Pitanguy, I.: Mamaplastias estudos de 245 casos consecutivos e apresentaçâo de tecnica pessoal. Rev. Bras. Cir. 42:201–220, 1961.

57. Pousson, M.: De la mastopexie. Bull. Soc. Chir. (Paris) 13:507–508, 1897.

58. Quervain (de), F.: Zur operativen Behandlung der Hängebrust. Zentralbl. Chir. 43:2423, 1925.

59. Ragnell, A.: Operative correction of hypertrophy and ptosis of the female breast. Acta Chir. Scand. [Suppl.] 113:13–149, 1946.

60. Regnault, P.: One hundred cases of the retromammary implantation of etheron, followed up for 30 months. Transactions of the Third International Congress of Plastic and Reconstructive Surgery, Washington, 1963. Excerpta Medica, Amsterdam, 1963, pp. 78–80.

61. Regnault, P.: In: Goldwyn, R. M. (ed.): Plastic and Reconstructive Surgery of the Breast. Boston, Little, Brown and Co., 1976.

62. Schrudde, J.: Eine Methode der Mammaplastik, Transacta der III Tagung der Vereinigung der Deutschen plastischen Chirurgen, Köln, 1972, pp. 89–91.

63. Schwarzman, E.: Über eine neue Methode der Mammaplastik. Wien. Med. Wochenschr. 86:100–102, 1936.

64. Skoog, T.: A technique of breast reduction. Acta Chir. Scand. 126:453–465, 1963.

65. Strombeck, J. O.: Mammaplasty: report of a new technique based on the two pedicle procedure. Br. J. Plast. Surg. 13:79–90, 1960.

66. Thorek, M.: Plastic Surgery of the Breast and Abdominal Wall. Charles C. Thomas, Springfield, Ill., 1942.

67. Velpeau, A.: Traité des Maladies du Sein et de la Région Mammaire. Masson et Cie, Paris, 1854.

68. Watson, J.: Some observations on free fat grafts: with reference to their use in mammaplasty. Br. J. Plast. Surg. 12:263–274, 1959.

69. Weiner, D. L., Aiache, A. E., Silver, L., and Tittiranonda, T.: A single dermal pedicle for nipple transposition in subcutaneous mastectomy, reduction mammaplasty, or mastopexy. Plast. Reconstr. Surg. 51:115–120, 1973.

70. Winkler, E.: Korrekturoperationen der weiblichen Brust. Zentralbl. Chir. 92:2007–2011, 1967.

The History of Abdominal Dermolipectomy

Paule Regnault M.D. F.R.C.S. (C)

Montreal, Canada

Until recently, the correction of abdominal wall deformities was restricted to the excess of adipose tissue with concomitant skin looseness and hernias (5–14).

The first attempt at classification was in 1931 by Passot (12) who classified the cases in *adipose abdominale généralisée* and *adipose abdominale sous ombilicale*.

But the differentiation between cases of excess fat and pure dermochalasis with no or little excess fat was stressed for the first time in Rio in 1971 with a proposed new technique restricted to the category of purely aesthetic motivation (13). The history of abdominal dermolipectomy is, therefore, the history of operations dealing with adipose aprons.

The first operation published on this subject seems to have been by Kelly (11) at the end of the nineteenth century (Fig. 1). Kelly claimed that he was the first one to have taken care of women with abdominal panniculus (John Hopkins, Baltimore, 1899). Kelly wrote: "I believe, that because the condition has been looked upon as natural, as well as inevitable and irremediable, it has thus far received so little attention." The operation described by Kelly was a horizontal wedge resection including the umbilicus. The technique was later described by Peters (Baltimore, 1901), who removed 7450 g from the abdomen of a 32-year-old woman. The piece removed was 90 cm long, 31 cm wide, and 7 cm thick. The umbilicus was situated at the center of the mass; no undermining was done.

A classification is necessary to clarify the history and evolution of the techniques published later. Three classes of techniques can be distinguished according to the direction of the excision and the resulting scar: the horizontal techniques, the vertical techniques, and the mixed techniques—using both vertical and horizontal directions at the same time.

Address reprint requests to Paule Regnault, M.D., La Tour de la Cité, P.O. Box 951, Montreal, H2W 2N1, Canada.

0364–216X/78/0002–0113 $02.20

© 1978 Springer-Verlag New York Inc.

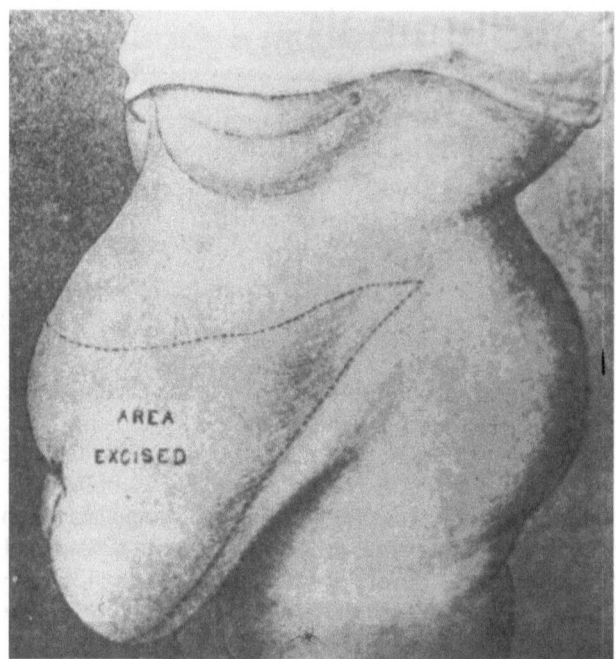

Fig. 1. Kelly resection published in *Johns Hopkins Med. J.* in 1899.

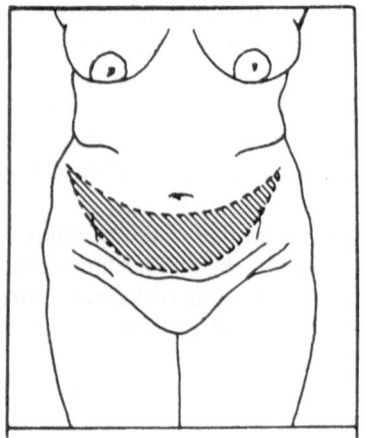

Fig. 2. Thorek operation, 1942.

Horizontal excisions

Following Kelly's operation, no other horizontal excision was described until Flesh-Thebesius and Wheisheimer (6) in 1931 removed the lower part of the abdominal adiposity as well as the umbilicus without any undermining. That same year Passot (12) described a lower horizontal excision with defatting up to the umbilicus.

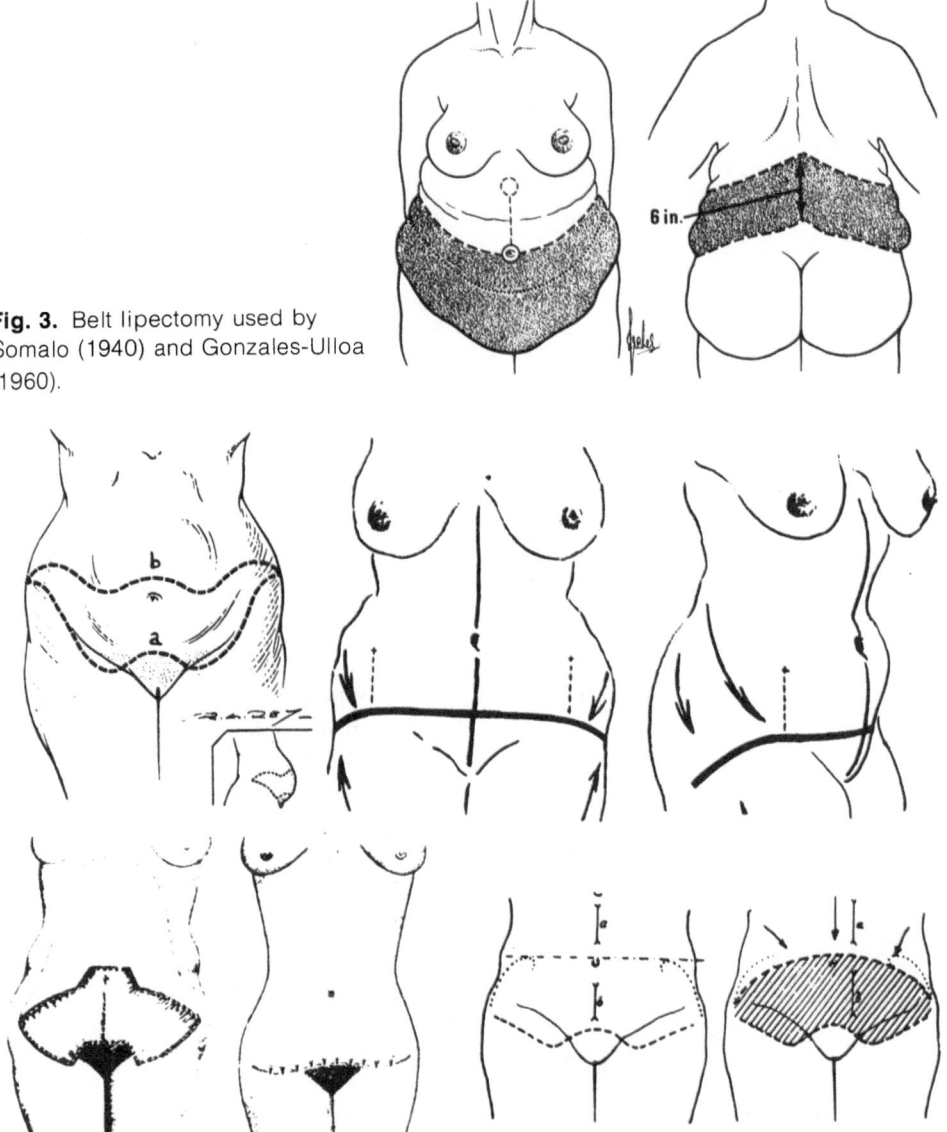

Fig. 3. Belt lipectomy used by Somalo (1940) and Gonzales-Ulloa (1960).

Fig. 4. Horizontal resections with extensive undermining and umbilical transposition. *Top:* (left to right: Spadafora, Pitanguy. *Bottom:* Serson, Callia.

In 1942 Thorek (22, 23) also removed the lower part of the abdominal skin and fat below the umbilicus, which was left intact, and without undermining (Fig. 2). Pick and Barsky (13) in 1949 proposed a modified Thorek technique with removal of wedges of tissue in the center and at the ends of the lower incision to prevent dog-ears.

The most important work later published on the subject was by Vernon (24) in

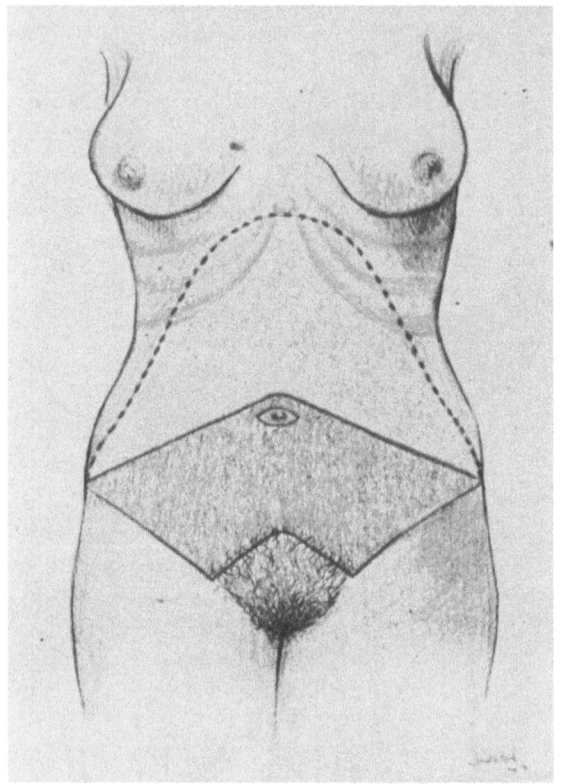

Fig. 5. W resection with extensive undermining indicated in abdomina dermochalasis without or with little excess fat tissue.

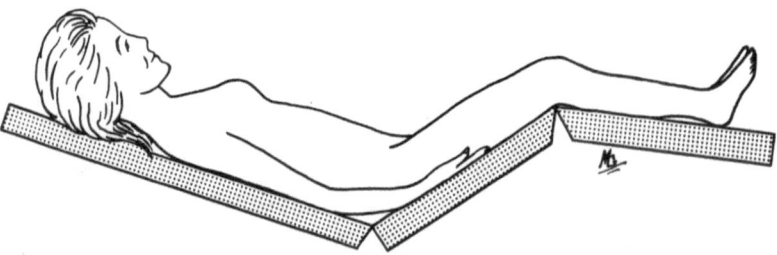

Fig. 6. Jackknife position of the operating table and bed.

1957: he was the first to describe the *transposition of the umbilicus,* with a horizontal excision of the lower abdominal panniculus, almost similar to the Thorek technique but undermining the upper part of the abdominal skin and fat. The umbilical incision was a circle and a similar circle was excised in the flap to locate the umbilicus. Although the same operation had already been done in Europe (by Dr. Noel), it had not been published before.

Somalo (20) in 1940 and Gonzalez-Ulloa (9) in 1960 proposed complete circular removal of the panniculus, a "belt" lipectomy (Fig. 3), with transposition of the

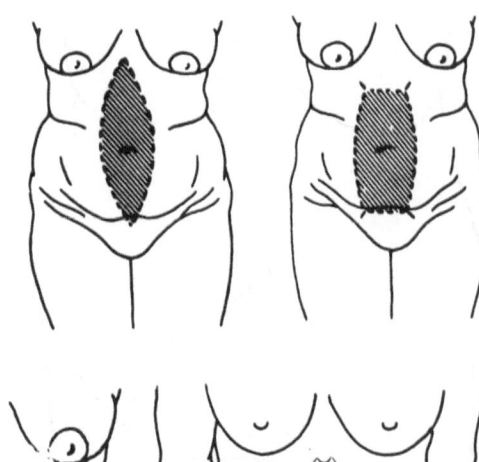

Fig. 7. Vertical excisions: Babcock (1916) and Kuster (1926).

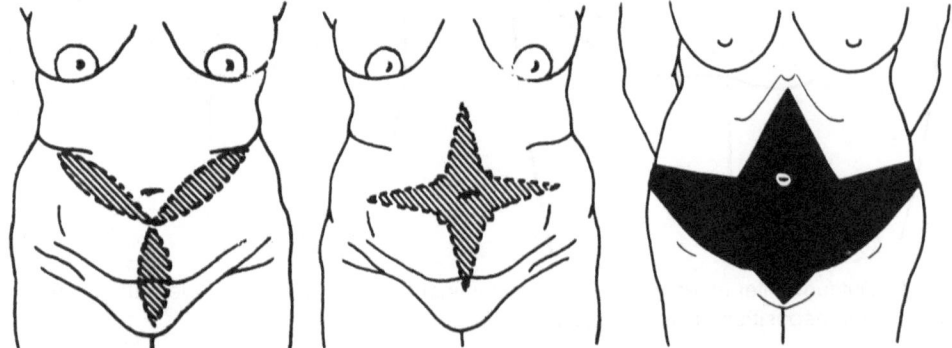

Fig. 8. Mixed resections with no undermining. *Left to right:* Weinhold (1909), Galtier (1955), Castanares and Goethel (1967).

umbilicus in the upper flap undermining moderately the middle part of the upper flap.

Spadafora (21) in 1962 removed the lower part of the abdominal apron with a horizontal sinusoidal excision, undermining the upper abdomen with a transposition of the umbilicus (Fig. 4). The Spadafora excision is located very high laterally above the iliac spines.

Pitanguy (14, 15) in 1967 proposed a horizontal excision located a little above the pubic hair and going downward laterally, doing an extensive undermining of the upper part of the abdomen and an umbilical transposition in the upper flap. Also in 1967 in the same country, Brasil, Callia (2), a general surgeon, published a low Spadafora-like sinusoidal excision of the lower abdomen including the upper part of the anterior portion of the thighs.

Serson (19) in 1971 presented a very low excision with an upper thigh, small extension, and two lateral small flaps in the upper part of the abdomen.

In 1972 Regnault (16, 17) published the W technique (Fig. 5). The excision's lower line is located in the upper part of pubic hair medially and follows the inguinal fold laterally. The upper line of the excision is straight oblique in the vertical position, becoming curved when the patient lies down. The principle of releasing the tissue at the midline while most tension is brought on the hips was shown for the

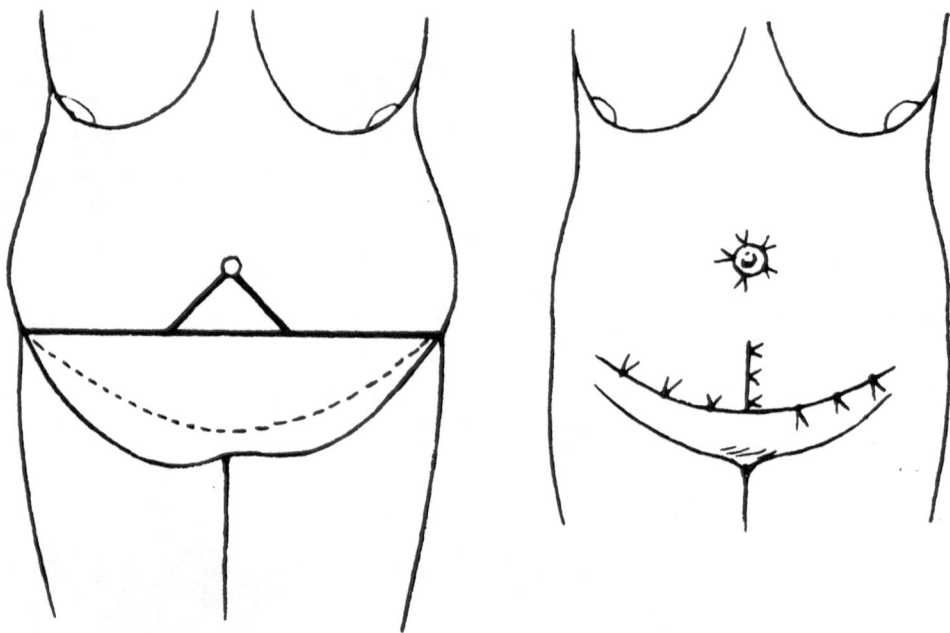

Fig. 9. Dufourmentel resection of lower abdominal fat with moderate undermining and umbilical transposition. Inverted T scar.

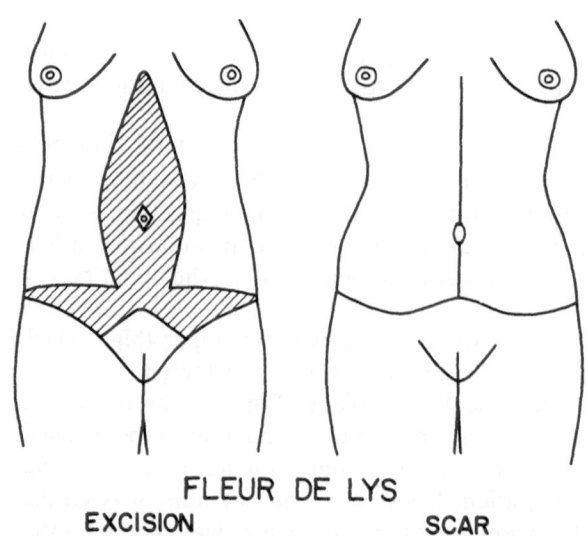

FLEUR DE LYS

EXCISION   SCAR

Fig. 10. *Fleur de lys* resection—mixed technique without undermining indicated in large low adiposity.

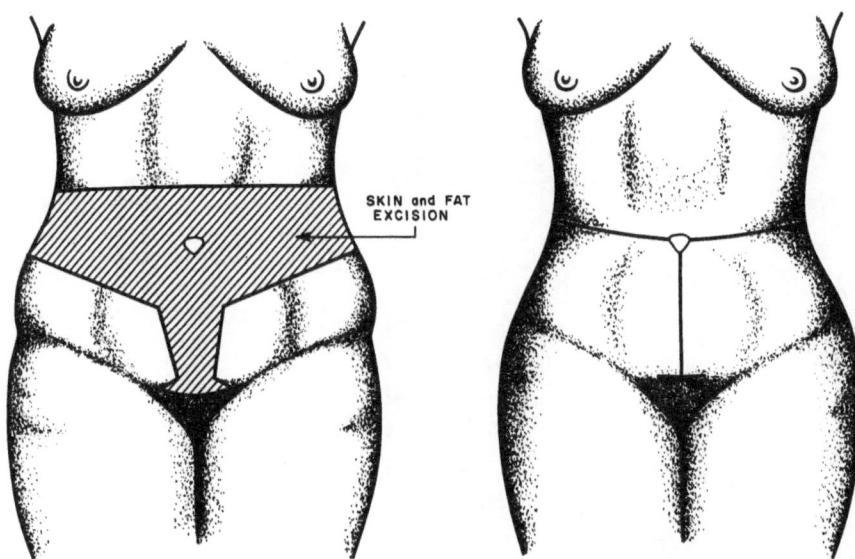

SKIN and FAT
EXCISION

Fig. 11. Belt lipectomy with lower abdominal vertical wedge with no or limited undermining indicated in large upper adiposity.

first time. The umbilicus is incised in a horizontal "marquise cut" shape, to be located in a horizontal incision in the upper flap. With the publication of this technique, the jackknife position of the patient on the table and in the bed was shown and stressed for the first time (Fig. 6).

Vertical excisions

The vertical technique was first demonstrated by Babcock (1) in 1916 (Fig. 7). It was a spindle-shaped excision at the midline from xyphoid to pubis sacrificing the umbilicus.

Schepelman (18) in 1918 proposed a similar excision with a wider removal of the lower abdominal tissues. Kuster in 1926 proposed a quadrangular vertical excision with small wedges at the four angles. It seems that no other vertical excision has been demonstrated since then.

Mixed techniques

In these techniques, the removal is in both vertical and horizontal directions. The first publication presenting such technique was by Weinhold (25) in 1909 (Fig. 8). He described an excision with three branches, each one having a spindle shape. One branch was at the lower mid portion of the lower abdomen. Two lateral symmetric branches were oblique, almost horizontal, joining with the upper end of the first lower incision. The umbilicus was kept in place; no undermining was done.

Passot (12) in 1931 proposed a local circular periumbilical excision keeping the

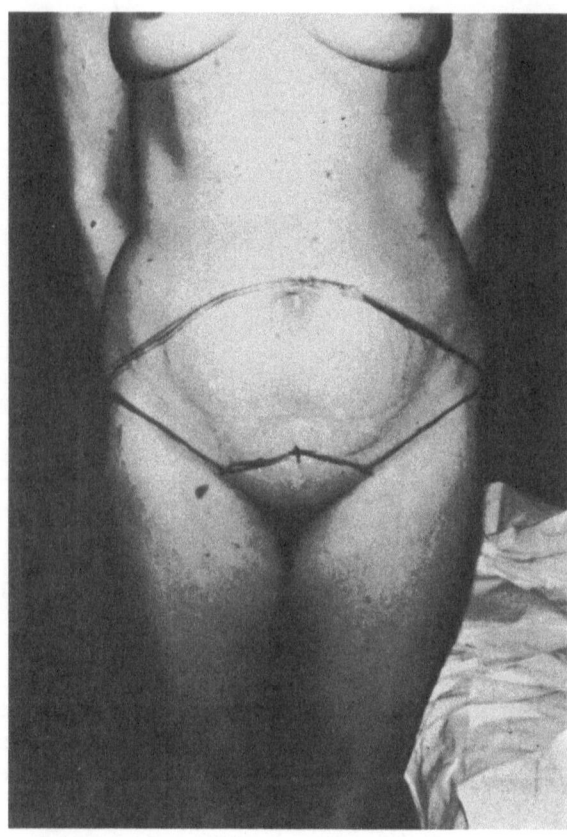

Fig. 12. (A) Typical case of W technique in a young woman with post-partum deformity; little fat.

umbilicus in place and closing with a "racket scar" (circle with a vertical component).

In 1955 Galtier (7) published a four wings star excision with the umbilicus as the center and kept in place. The scar was like a cross with the umbilicus at the center. No undermining was done. Long before, Morestin, who is mentioned in Passot's book, had performed the same type of excision but sacrificing the umbilicus. It was criticized by Passot as "rather an operation for orthopedists than for esthetic surgeons," giving excellent weight reduction but bad scars with "an inevitable resection of the umbilicus."

In 1959 Dufourmentel and Mouly (4) published a mixed technique removing the lower part of the abdomen with a vertical wedge in the upper part and a moderate undermining (Fig. 9). The umbilicus was transposed in the upper flap. The resulting scar was an inverted T, the vertical branch more or less remaining away from the umbilicus. Lately, F. Grazer (10) has published a similar technique.

In 1967 Castanares and Goethel published a modified Galtier technique, the four branches of the excision being unequal and the whole excision removing more tissue horizontally than vertically. The resulting scar is also a cross, the umbilicus located in the vertical upper scar.

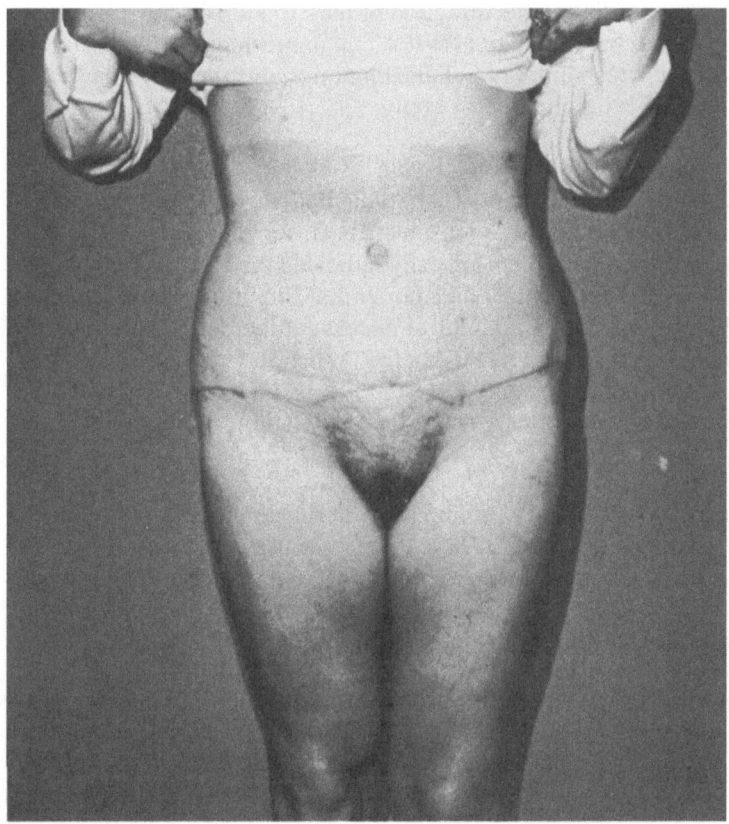

Fig. 12. (B) Typical result after 1 year. Note waistline and umbilicus location.

In 1975 Regnault (17) published two mixed techniques. The first is the *fleur de lys* excision (Fig. 10), which is a modified Castanares technique, the excision having three branches, one vertical and two lateral. The lower incision is in a W shape respecting the pubic area. The second technique (Fig. 11), presented in the same publication, is also a three-branched excision, modified belt lipectomy, with a vertical component and without undermining but with the umbilicus at the center of the excision and at the center of the resulting scar. Two small wedges at the lower end permit resection of the monte veneri. No undermining is done. The final scar has a T shape.

Present classification

In light of the past management of abdominal lipectomies, a classification was published by Dufourmentel and Mouly (4), who proposed to classify these cases in two categories: cases with hernias or diastasis of the muscles and cases of simple adiposity.

Later a classification according to the direction of the excision (16) was proposed which has just been studied here. Today (17) it seems more logical to classify the cases in three categories corresponding to clinical findings and therefore deducting the right indication of the best technique to apply.

First category

This category includes cases with a thick abdominal layer. Most of the patients are older women with concomitant large muscular diastases or hernias.

In these cases, the surgical techniques logically indicated are those permitting the largest possible removal in both vertical and horizontal directions without undermining of tissues. When the greatest amount of excess fat lies at the lower part of the abdomen, the *fleur de lys* operation is indicated. When the greatest amount lies at the upper part of the abdomen, the T technique, sometimes extended to a semicircular belt lipectomy if necessary, is the best indication.

Second category

The second category includes post-partum cases, dermochalasis, and those who have experienced a great loss of weight. The patients are usually younger women. The diastasis of the recti often must be corrected. In these cases the resulting scar should remain in an easily concealed area, just above the pubic hair. The techniques therefore indicated are those using an extensive undermining with umbilical transposition and good traction over the hips (Fig. 12). The W technique is the most logical: it brings good aesthetic result with little morbidity. Occasionally a young woman with thick adiposity wants a low horizontal scar. The W may be used but the volume reduction cannot be as drastic as with a mixed technique.

Third category

Intermediate cases are included in the third category. Some cases with various scars and localized excess tissue do not fall in these two categories. They may present various problems due to the number of the scars, their location, the location of the excess tissue. Most of the time they require a scar excision with moderate undermining and conversion of vertical scars into horizontal ones if possible.

Conclusion

Abdominal dermolipectomies were performed almost a century ago. The procedure was a simple one-direction excision without undermining. The more elaborate techniques of today have been developed over several decades. The main step has been the umbilical transposition, published in 1957 by Vernon (24).

The classification in two main categories of techniques according to the case seems to be an important step in this matter. The principle of releasing tension in the midline by stretching tissues laterally as well as innovations in the position of the patient have brought great benefit in the treatment of abdominal lipodystrophy and dermochalasis.

References

1. Babcock, W.: Plastic reconstruction of the female breasts and abdomen. Am. J. Surg. 43:260, 1939.

2. Callia, W. E. B.: Una plastica para o cirurgia geral. Med. Hosp. (Sao Paulo) 1:40–41, 1967.

3. Castanares, S., and Goethel, J.: Abdominal lipectomy: a modification in technique. Plast. Reconstr. Surg. 40:378–383, 1967.

4. Dufourmentel, C., and Mouly, R.: Chirurgie Plastique. Flammarion et Cie, Paris, 1959, pp. 381–389.

5. Edgerton, M. Y. T., and Knor, N. J.: Motivational patterns of patients seeking cosmetic (esthetic) surgery. Plast. Reconstr. Surg. 48:551–557, 1971.

6. Flesch-Thebesius, M., and Wheisheimer, K.: Die Operation des Hängebauches. Chirurgie 3:841, 1931.

7. Galtier, W.: Obésité de la paroi abdominale. Presse Méd. 70:135, 1962.

8. Serson, D.: Geometric planning for abdominal dermolipectomy. In: Year Book of Plastic and Reconstructive Surgery, 1972. Chicago, Year Book Medical Publishing Co., 1973, pp. 132–134.

9. Gonzalez-Ulloa, M.: Belt lipectomy. Br. J. Plast. Reconstr. Surg. 13: 1960.

10. Grazer, F. M.: Abdominoplasty. Plast. Reconstr. Surg. 51:617–623, 1973.

11. Kelly, H. A.: Johns Hopkins Med. J. 10:197, 1899.

12. Passot, R.: Chirurgie Esthétique Pure. G. Doin, Editeur, Paris, 1931, pp. 261–267.

13. Pick, J. F.: Surgery of Repair, Vol. 2. J.B. Lippincott Co., Philadelphia, 1949, p. 445.

14. Pitanguy, I.: Abdominal lipectomy: an approach to it through an analysis of 300 consecutive cases. Plast. Reconstr. Surg. 40:383–391, 1967.

15. Pitanguy, I.: Technique for trunk and thigh reductions. In: Transactions of the 5th International Congress for Plastic and Reconstructive Surgery. Butterworths, Sydney, Australia, pp. 1204–1210.

16. Regnault, P.: Abdominal dermolipectomy. Internat. Microfilm. J. Aesthet. Plast. Surg., 1972. (Dr. J. Tamerin, 44 E. 67 St., N.Y., N.Y.)

17. Regnault, P.: Abdominal dermolipectomies. Clin. Plast. Surg. 2(3):411–429, 1975.

18. Shepelman, E.: Ueber Bauchdeckenplastik mit besonderer Beachtung des Hängebauches. Beitr. Klin. Chir. 3:372, 1918.

19. Serson, D.: Planeamento geometrico. La dema lypectomia abdominal. Rev. Esp. Cir. Plast. 4:37–42, 1971.

20. Somalo, M.: Dermolipectomia circular del tronco. Sem. Med. I:1435–1443, 1940.

21. Spadafora, A.: Abdomen pendulo, dermolipectomia antero lateral baya. Prensa Med. Argent. 49:494–499, 1962.

22. Thoreck, P.: Anatomy in Surgery. Philadelphia, J.B. Lippincott Co., 1951, pp. 363–397.

23. Thorek, M.: Plastic reconstruction of the female breasts and abdomen. Am. J. Surg. 43:268–278, 1939.

24. Vernon, S.: Umbilical transplantation upward and abdominal contouring in lipectomy. Am. J. Surg. 94:490–492, 1957.

25. Weinhold, S.: Bauchdeckenplastik. Zentralbl Gynaekol. 38:1332, 1909.